# 10-MINUTE STRETCHING

# 10-MINUTE STRETCHING

## Simple Exercises to Build Flexibility into Your Daily Routine

HILERY HUTCHINSON

ILLUSTRATIONS BY CHRISTY NI

ROCKRIDGE PRESS

For general information on our other products and services or to obtain technical support, please contact our Customer Care Department within the United States at (866) 744-2665, or outside the United States at (510) 253-0500.

Rockridge Press publishes its books in a variety of electronic and print formats. Some content that appears in print may not be available in electronic books, and vice versa.

Interior and Cover Designer: Michael Cook
Photo Art Director/Art Manager: Sara Feinstein
Editor: Mo Mozuch
Production Editor: Ashley Polikoff

Illustration © 2020 Christy Ni. All other art used under license from iStock.com.

ISBN: Print 978-1-6473-9738-8 | eBook 978-1-6473-9440-0

R0

# Contents

*In loving memory of Ernest A. Hutchinson Jr.*
*Thank you for being my daily inspiration*
*to help people on their journey to wellness.*

# Introduction

Stretching is simple, it's free, you can do it anywhere, it requires no equipment, and it has the power to transform lives. How cool is that?

My curiosity for stretching started when I was a six-year-old girl trying to get my splits for gymnastics class. I would spend hours practicing them and even did my homework sitting in splits. It wasn't until I became a personal trainer in my early twenties that I really started to study the subject and understand flexibility on a deeper level beyond my firsthand experience. I quickly learned how a lack of flexibility limits us in a variety of ways and takes a toll not only on our lifestyle, but also our health and pain levels. Tight muscles result in both injuries and poor posture that can lead to health issues, balance problems, and further injuries. For our bodies to operate in their peak state, they must be flexible.

The effect that flexibility levels have on our daily lives is what really inspired me to invest so much time in learning more. I decided to make flexibility the focus of my career in fitness and wellness because of how good the success stories make me feel. It's always nice when a client hits their goal weight, but it is a whole different level of feel-good vibes when a client's entire quality of life changes. I am elated when I get a message from a client celebrating a hike with their grandkids for the first time or doing some home repair projects with ease because they have better mobility, stamina, and balance from their stretching practice. It excites me when stretching takes away pain in a client's joints and muscles or helps an athlete perform better and recover faster. I think it is amazing how stretching can make everyday tasks easier no matter what age you are, and it takes very little time to see results.

I'm hoping that by writing this book I will be able to help even more people gain the benefits of stretching. This book will help you learn everything you need to know about safe and effective stretching, including how flexibility works and its benefits. Step-by-step directions for 60 individual stretches are accompanied by illustrations and alternative ways to make the stretches accessible to all body types and mobility levels. Then you will learn 35 essential stretching routines that can all be done in 10 minutes or less, with tips on how to breathe and perform each sequence. These routines are designed to supplement everyday activities, athletic endeavors, injury rehab, and pain relief. Finally, you will learn how to create your own unique routines that are both safe and effective.

Stretching routines do not take a lot of time and the rewards are very gratifying. All of the routines in this book can be done in less than 10 minutes. Consistency is the key to getting results, so make sure you sneak stretching routines into your day whenever you can! Most of my clients notice a difference after just a week of stretching, so it won't take very long to see and feel the benefits.

# Glossary

active stretching: Holding a position using the muscle you are focused on with no other support.

all-fours position: Coming down to your hands and knees with your wrists lined up under your shoulders and knees directly below your hips.

anterior: The front side of the body.

box breathing: Making your breath equal parts inhaling, holding your breath in, exhaling, and holding your breath out. For example: Inhale for five seconds, hold your breath in for five seconds, exhale for five seconds, and hold your breath out for five seconds.

contraction: Engaging a muscle.

contraindication: A factor or reason that you should not perform an exercise.

dynamic stretching: Quick movements that warm up the body and prepare it for movement.

fascia: Connective tissue that runs through every part of your body like a spiderweb.

flexibility: The ability of each of your joints to move through their full range of motion.

isometric stretching: Holding a stretch while engaging the muscle.

indication: A factor or reason to perform an exercise.

passive stretching: Using an external force to help you go deeper into a stretch.

proprioceptive neuromuscular facilitation (PNF): A technique discovered by physical therapists to contract a muscle while stretching in an effort to get a deeper stretch.

posterior: The back side of the body.

proprioception: Knowing where your body is in space.

resistance stretching: Passing through a full range of motion in a stretch while applying resistance.

static stretching: Staying still and holding a stretch.

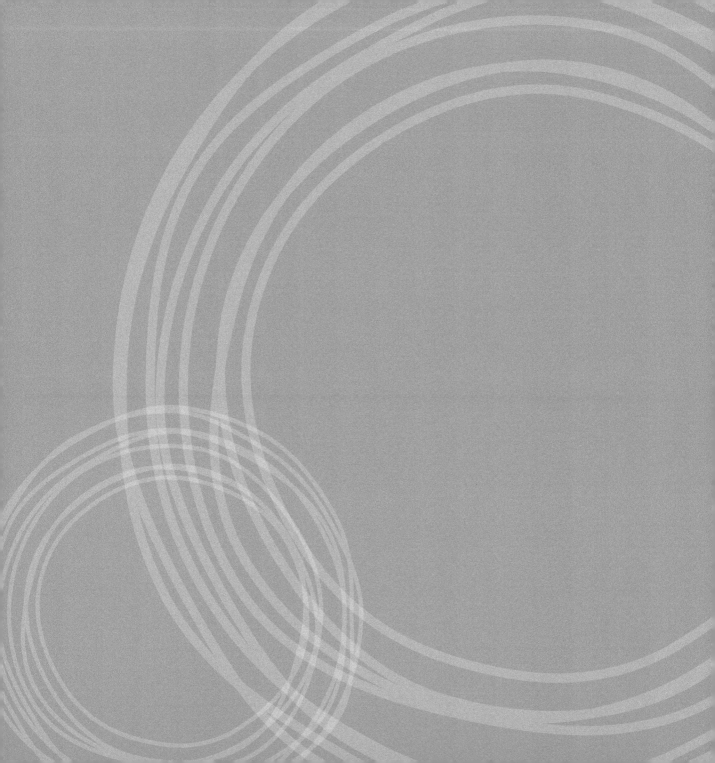

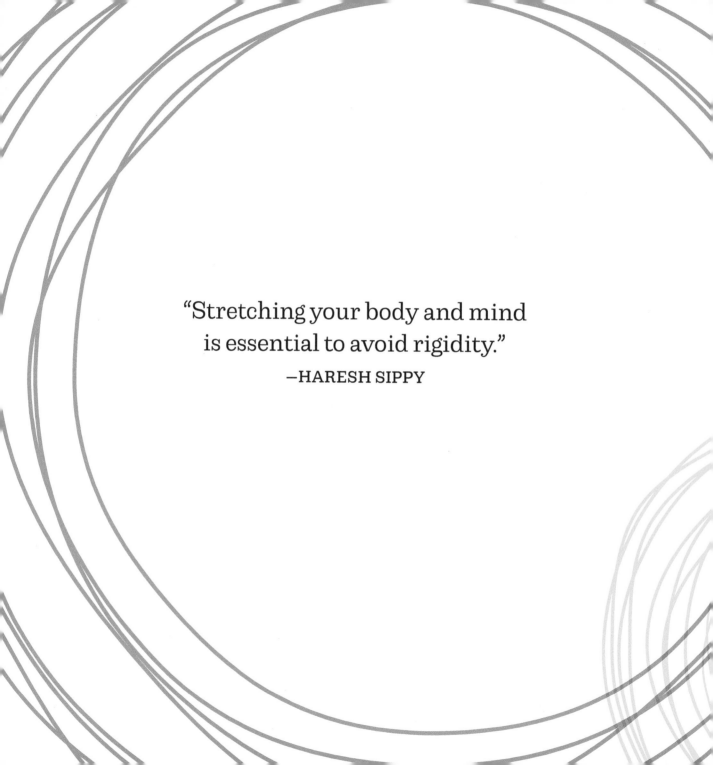

"Stretching your body and mind
is essential to avoid rigidity."

—HARESH SIPPY

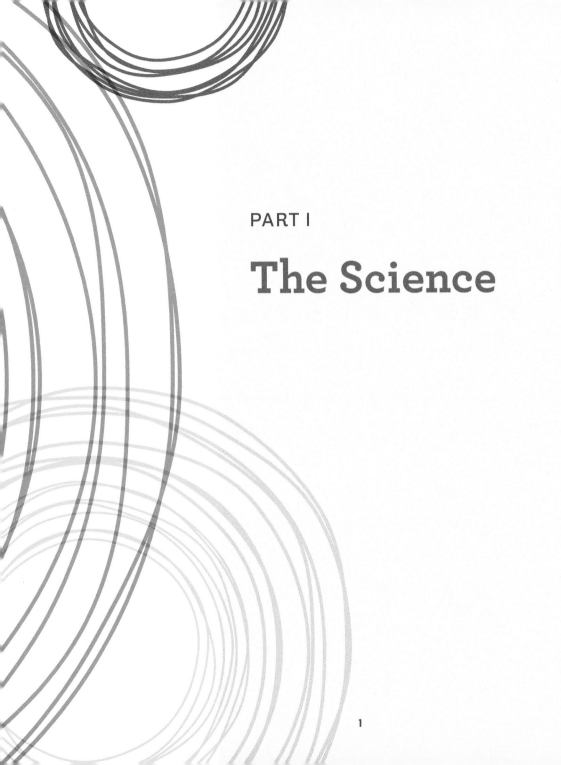

PART I

# The Science

Stretching feels amazing! We all naturally stretch a little here and there, whether we're yawning or bending over to put our shoes on. Stretching is often considered a form of physical exercise, but I like to think of it as a completely natural way to move your body as it truly desires.

As our bodies age and we experience life, posture issues, injuries, and diminishing mobility often occur. I think many people succumb and assume this is just part of aging, but I'm here to inform you that there is hope. Stretching can solve all of these issues, and it is never too late to start.

Proper stretching takes such a short amount of time and only requires a little bit of knowledge about how flexibility works and what stretches to do in order to solve your problems and achieve your goals.

Improper stretching happens when you aren't listening to your body. You never want to force your body to work through pain or bounce using momentum during a stretch. It is vital to know the difference between proper and improper stretching in order to stay safe and avoid injury.

Part I of this book will provide you with everything you need to know about how flexibility and stretching work, the benefits stretching provides, and the different types of stretching you can do. You will be amazed at how simple stretching is and how profound the benefits are.

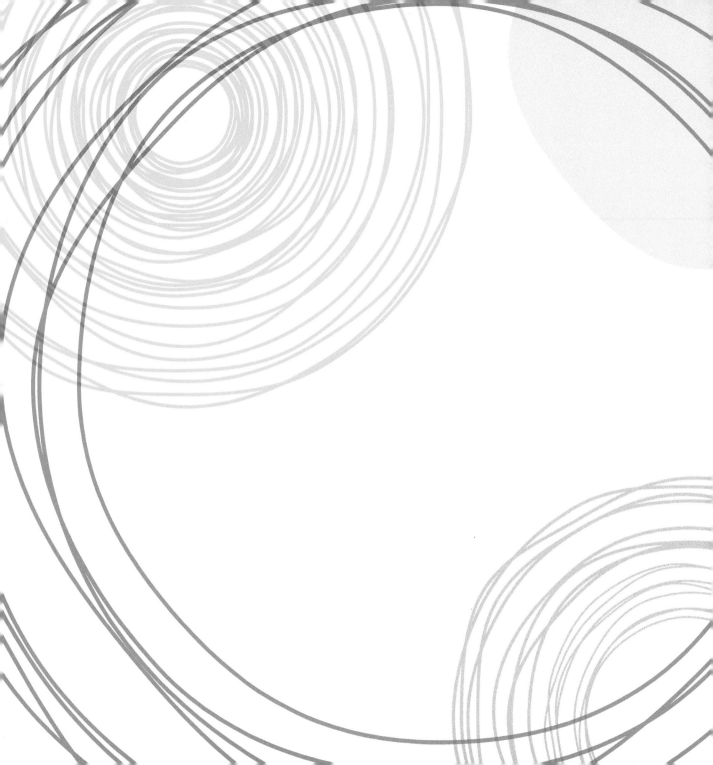

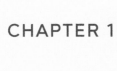

CHAPTER 1

# Why Stretching Works

How well do you know your muscles? This is important information to understand, as it will help you have the most effective stretching sessions.

Did you know that there are 650 skeletal muscles in the body, or that your tongue alone is controlled by eight different muscles? Our muscles help us do everything in life, from taking a shower to lifting heavy objects. All muscles are made of the same material even though they are different shapes and sizes and have different functions. Muscle tissue is very elastic, like a rubber band, so that it can easily move, contract, and stretch. Each muscle we have is made up of thousands of small individual muscle fibers.

Muscle cells contain two different protein filaments: actin and myosin. These filaments slide past one another to produce a contraction that changes the shape and length of the muscle cells. There's actually a tiny chemical reaction going on in your muscles every time you move. Our muscles are attached to the bones by tendons—tough bands of connective tissue made from collagen. This gives each muscle in our body a distinct purpose to help move our bones and joints in a very particular way.

We have two different defense mechanisms built into our muscles to protect us from overstretching: muscle spindles and the Golgi tendon organ. Muscle spindles run all through the muscle fibers, sensing the rate of change in length, and they cause muscles to contract in an effort to protect you from pulling a muscle. The Golgi tendon organ is found in the tendons, and as it senses the rate of change in tension, it tells muscles to relax in an effort to protect the tendons. Knowing this helps us understand that it is better to slowly move into a stretch rather than immediately pushing yourself to your limit.

Muscles need to be stretched in order to keep them flexible and healthy. Without stretching, our muscles naturally become shorter and tighter over time. The less active you are, the tighter things become. Life is so much easier when your body can move freely without limitations and restrictions! The more frequently you stretch, the more flexibility you gain. This flexibility helps you out in all of your daily activities and improves your overall health and quality of life.

There are several different factors that can contribute to how flexible you are:

Joint Structure — The structure of your joints can limit your flexibility. The hip joint is a perfect example of this. Your hip joint looks like a ball and socket. The ball can be inserted into the socket at three slightly different positions, depending on the specific anatomy you were born with. One of these positions means you will never be able to achieve a straddle split because the bones just aren't capable of that range of motion.

Age — As our bodies age, they go through a slow dehydration process. As we lose water in our body, we lose elasticity in our muscles and tendons, which results in feeling stiff. Your age does not mean you can't make progress, though.

Gender — Women are naturally more flexible than men, regardless of age, because of their joint structure. While pregnant, females increase their levels of a hormone called relaxin, making their bodies even more flexible.

Injuries and Surgeries — When we are injured, our bodies heal and repair by a process called fibrosis. This can create scar tissue, dense fascia, and adhesions that can limit our full range of motion.

Posture — Over time, posture is manipulated by your muscles. As muscles become tighter, they pull on the bones, forcing your body into a more restricted position. This restricted position will also limit other ranges of motion. Other posture issues that affect flexibility due to curvature of the spine are kyphosis, lordosis, and scoliosis.

Muscle Mass — Big muscles can limit your ability to move through a full range of motion. Think about a bodybuilder with really large chest and back muscles. Those muscles can become so large that they restrict the full movement of the shoulders and arms.

Opposing Muscles — A muscle can lengthen only as much as the opposing muscle can contract, or shorten. For example, if you are trying to stretch your quadricep, but your hamstring can't contract as much as your quadricep can lengthen, then your flexibility in the quadricep is limited by your hamstring.

Another factor that plays a role is genetics. There are natural-born flexible people, but their flexibility tends to be caused by a genetic hypermobility condition. Not everyone has the potential to become a contortionist, even if you put in the time and effort.

One more thing we need to factor into how our muscles work is fascia, a type of connective tissue made of collagen that holds each organ, blood vessel, bone, nerve fiber, and muscle in place. Bob Cooley, author of *Resistance Flexibility 1.0*, compares fascia to soup stock, "...with muscles, tendons, bones, ligaments, etc. analogous to carrots, celery, potatoes, etc. within the soup. And like the soup broth, the fascia penetrates into the vegetables besides having its own layers. Thus, affecting the fascia dramatically affects all other tissues."

Fascia doesn't have any nerves, so it can't create pain itself, but it can accumulate and become denser, which restricts the ability of our muscles to function at their full capacity and can also reduce flexibility and mobility. We have to take care of our fascia if we want to be able to move with ease.

Have you ever noticed how you feel stiffer when you wake up in the morning than you do at the end of the day? This is because the less you move, the more crystal-like the fascia becomes; the more you move, the more liquid it becomes. Lying still for eight hours at night makes it start to congeal and crystalize. This is why issues like plantar fasciitis are much worse first thing in the morning. Stretching, foam rolling, massage, and staying hydrated are all ways to help improve the health of our fascia.

# The Benefits of Stretching

Static, dynamic, and proprioceptive neuromuscular facilitation (PNF) stretching have all been measured as successful stretching modalities to improve flexibility, but most research studies have noted an individualized response to stretching. This means it is important to customize your stretching routine to what feels best in your body. Talk with your doctor or physical therapist about the best stretches for any of your concerns.

A simple, short stretch routine has a multitude of benefits, and when done regularly, those benefits are compounded. You may feel like you were just born tight and may find it hard to believe that simple stretching could be just as beneficial as bendy positions in a yoga class, but no matter what your range of motion while stretching, the benefits are equal for everyone.

I feel like the benefits of stretching could fill an entire chapter of this book! My clients are always amazed when they can reach their toes and sit comfortably on the floor for the first time. Then they begin to see how that flexibility improves different aspects of their lives. Here are the eight common benefits of stretching:

Pain Relief — Stretching is a natural pain reliever on a few different levels. It increases your circulation, which can help injuries heal quicker; it stretches tight muscles that are pulling on the joints and creating pain; and it releases endorphins like dopamine that help you feel good.

Increased Flexibility — A flexible body makes everyday routines such as getting dressed or working around the house easier to accomplish. Our flexibility levels naturally decrease with age, but with stretching, we can reverse this process and stay mobile for years to come.

Increased Circulation — By stretching your muscles, you are also stretching your blood vessels. This helps improve circulation and blood flow throughout the day.

Boosted Energy Levels — Your energy levels naturally increase in response to stretching because of improved circulation and increased endorphins.

Improved Posture — Poor posture is a result of one muscle being too tight and the opposing muscle becoming weak. Every posture correction plan uses a combination of stretching and strengthening to bring the body into balance.

Stress Relief — Stress naturally causes our muscles to tense up. It is part of the fight-or-flight response. Through stretching and deep breathing we are able to put our nervous system into the rest-and-digest phase, when our muscles naturally relax while our stress levels decrease.

Injury Prevention — Stretching keeps the muscles long and supple so that they can move through all your different ranges of motion with ease. Keeping the muscles supple is the best way to prevent injuries like a pulled muscle or to protect you from falls.

Enhanced Coordination and Balance — Stretching increases your level of proprioception, and because your body is more mobile, it can react more quickly in terms of both balance and coordination. Lower body stretching helps reduce the risk of falls.

## Why 10 Minutes

I have been working with clients on flexibility for 18 years. During this time, I have run a lot of different experiments to see what is most effective in increasing flexibility quickly. When it comes to the amount of time you need to stretch, I've found that doing two 10-minute sessions a week is enough time to *significantly* increase the overall flexibility of my senior clients in just six weeks.

Recent research shows that stretching for just five minutes a day, five days a week, can help improve your range of motion. A 10-minute routine is the perfect length to seriously improve your flexibility and make a wide variety of activities more enjoyable.

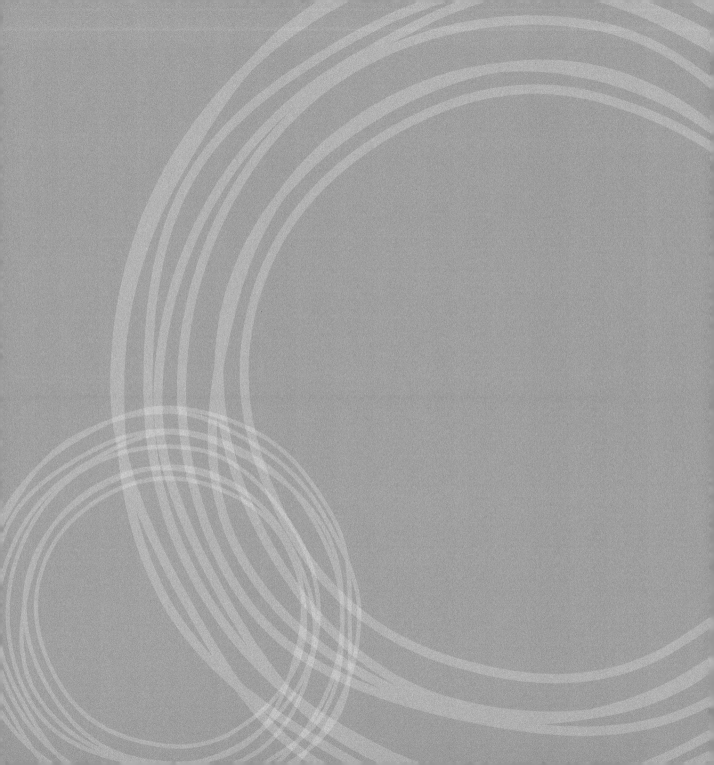

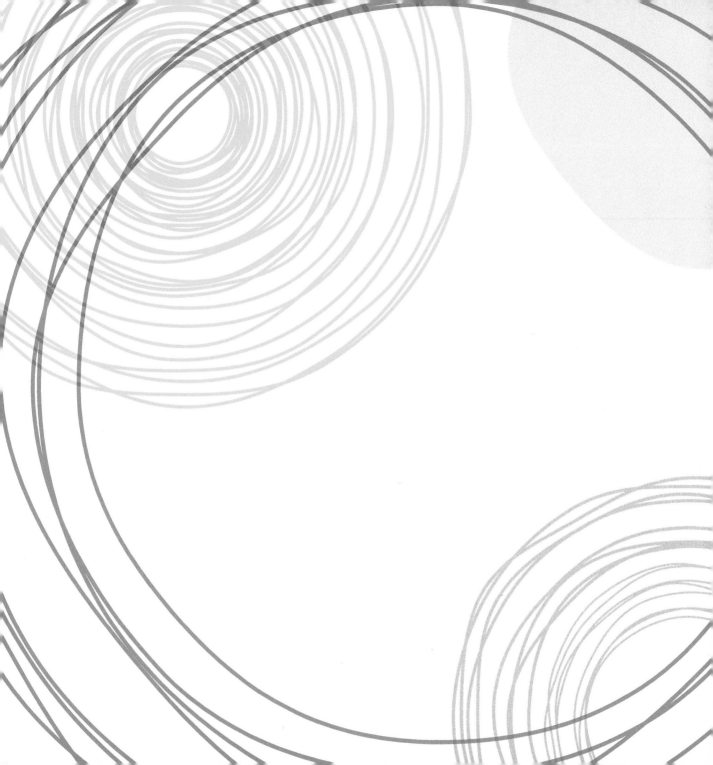

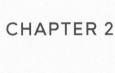

## CHAPTER 2

# Proper Stretching Techniques

Step one of setting up a stretching routine is finding a space for it. It is important that you have enough room to move freely without feeling constricted. Stretching can be done anywhere, so selecting a space is really about your comfort. It is best to stretch when warm, so I would not recommend having the air conditioning on or doing it outside in cold weather without warming up your body first.

# Clear Your Mind

Before you stretch, it is always a good idea to take a moment to check in with your body. I prefer to do this lying down on my back, but you can do it seated too. I encourage you to start by taking a few deep breaths and then notice how your body is sitting or lying on the floor. Are you perfectly straight? Is there more pressure on your right or left side? Does anything feel out of alignment? Then, mentally scan your body from the toes up to the crown of your head. Identify any areas that are in pain or muscles that feel like they are tense. Then you will have a much better idea of what needs to be stretched. I also check in with my mind just to be aware of how my mood shifts from stretching.

# What Makes a Good Stretch?

It is important to follow these five keys to get the most out of each and every stretch.

**Alignment:** A good stretch starts with the position of your bones. Make sure you not only look at the illustrations for each stretch but also read the directions and tips to help you understand the proper alignment. Always think about starting the movement of a stretch with a nice long spine, and then you can relax and soften into it.

## PNF STRETCHING

PNF stretching is short for proprioceptive neuromuscular facilitation and is one of the most effective forms of flexibility training to increase range of motion. In PNF we temporarily contract the target, or opposing muscle that we are stretching. This stimulates the Golgi tendon organ, which signals the muscle to relax. This creates length in the muscle that we can use by going deeper into the stretch. This is known in physiology as the "relaxation response."

The indications and contraindications for PNF stretching are similar to those of any type of stretching. Indications include a loss of range of motion, acute pain, chronic pain, muscle tightness, muscle cramps, and a lack of flexibility in the involved area.

Contraindications for PNF stretching include instability of a joint or area, age (18 and under), recent surgery, and already stretched muscles using the PNF technique. It is not good to perform PNF stretching more than once a day due to the amount of stress it places on muscles and tendons.

PNF stretching has three methods that you can apply to different stretches. These techniques are often done with a partner because it is difficult to push against stretches in certain positions. You can perform PNF techniques several times in a row until you stop seeing progress.

### Hold-Relax

1. Hold a passive stretch for 10 seconds.
2. Push against the stretch for 6 seconds. This is an isometric hold, meaning you are pushing and resisting against the stretch but you are not moving.
3. Relax into a passive stretch for 30 seconds.

### Contract-Relax

1. Hold a passive stretch for 10 seconds.
2. Push against the stretch through the full range of motion you took to get into the stretch.
3. Relax back into a passive stretch for 30 seconds.

### Contract-Relax with Agonist Contract

1. Hold a passive stretch for 10 seconds.
2. Push against the stretch isometrically for 10 seconds, then squeeze the opposing muscle for 10 seconds.
3. Relax back into a passive stretch for 30 seconds.

**Breathing:** Many times I see people hold their breath while stretching. You have to breathe! Many stretches can force you into a different breathing pattern. Some stretches can expand the lungs, helping you take deep breaths, while some constrict the lungs, forcing you to exhale further. You can follow the natural breathing patterns, but some people can have a difficult time connecting to these subtle shifts. If you would prefer to follow a specific breathing method, I recommend inhaling for four counts and exhaling for six counts.

**Isolation:** It is better to focus on one muscle group at a time while stretching. You will notice a difference in the intensity if you are focused on stretching one leg rather than both legs. By isolating a single muscle group, you will have better awareness and control to perform the stretch properly and effectively.

**Leverage:** Using leverage can make it easier to overcome the resistance and tension of tight muscles. Props (see page 18) can be very helpful in increasing your leverage in a stretch. A strap is one of the handiest tools for this, but I have also chosen stretches for this book that have the best leverage and positioning for this purpose.

**Timing:** The magic ingredient in the stretching equation is time. Unfortunately everyone's body is completely different, so there really is no magic number when it comes to how long to hold a stretch. Instead, I want you to pay attention to when you relax into a stretch. You want to wait for this magical moment of surrender. Your body has stopped fighting the stretch, and all of a sudden, it feels softer. This is the moment you are waiting for. If you can hold the stretch for about five deep breaths after this moment, it will do wonders to increase your flexibility.

The biggest risk associated with stretching is pulling a muscle, but that is an ailment nobody needs to suffer from! To keep your body safe, make sure you warm up properly, move slowly into your stretches, and don't bounce or use momentum.

# Warming Up and Cooling Down

It is super important to make sure you are warmed up before you stretch. I don't want you to feel like you need to run a race first. Instead, you can simply do some dynamic stretches as a warm-up. One of the benefits of dynamic stretching is that it increases range of motion without decreasing power. It is best to start with simple movements first and then try some more complex movements. If you are looking for stretches to do as a warm-up, try using these:

- Leg Swings (page 152)
- Hip Circles (page 120)
- Shoulder Circles (page 50)
- Arm Swings (page 60)

Stretching is generally used as a cooldown, so as long as you are not doing a dynamic stretch, it will be slowing your body down. Try using static stretches that are done while seated or lying down and feel more restful as a way to end your session. Here are a few suggestions to try at the end of your session:

- Fish (page 108)
- Seated Forward Fold (page 130)
- Supine Twist (page 98)
- Banana (page 104)

# Breathing

Your body will naturally know how to breathe in a stretch. Listen to it. Certain stretches will make you exhale more, while others will expand your lungs and help you take fuller breaths. Pay attention to how your breathing naturally changes in response to a stretch and work with it. If you would like to try a breathing technique that will help you deepen a stretch, just make sure you exhale longer than you inhale. This relaxes the nervous system and also helps relieve pain, allowing you to go deeper into a stretch.

# Counting

Everyone will have to listen to their body when assessing how long to hold a stretch. If you are very tight and just getting started, you may want to only hold a stretch for 20 seconds, switch sides, and repeat for another 20 seconds. If you are able to hold a stretch for longer, do it. You can set a timer on your phone for how long you want to hold a stretch, or you could try counting for a number of slow deep breaths. Try holding a stretch for five deep breaths or more, and it will help you be mindful of your breathing and gain deeper levels of stress relief while stretching.

# Props

Props can be extremely helpful because they can make a stretch more comfortable or give you better leverage. In my own practice, I have found that props help people deepen a stretch, but I think people often try to get by without them because they feel like they're a crutch. I will suggest different props to try in different stretches in part II, but this is how each type of prop tends to be the most helpful:

**Straps** are used as a way to make your arms longer and give yourself better leverage. You will often use a strap by wrapping it around your foot in order to reach farther. Think of straps as an extension of your arms.

**Blocks** are great for support. If you can't reach the floor, then add a couple of blocks and place your hands on them instead. You can place a block under your upper back, in between your shoulder blades, to support you in Fish pose (page 108) too.

**Chairs** can be used to help modify a stretch. If you are reaching down for the floor and it seems very far away, place a chair in front of yourself and reach for the seat. If you are doing a Standing Quad Stretch (page 126) and can't reach your foot, you could place your knee on the seat of a chair instead. You can also use a chair to help yourself balance better in certain stretches.

**Pillows** create comfort. If you are sitting with your legs in front of you and can't reach your toes, stacking a couple pillows on your lap can make a major difference in how comfortable the stretch is. I encourage you to get creative with your pillows!

**Foam rollers** can be used in a variety of ways when stretching. If you stand it up, it works just like a block. You could also place one under a joint or body part for more support—for instance, resting the back of your neck on it as you are working on your neck stretches.

**Blankets** can be rolled and folded in different ways to make stretches more comfortable. You may want to place one under your knee for extra cushioning or roll one up to provide extra support.

## Myths and Mistakes

**If you were born tight, there is no hope.** This couldn't be further from the truth! Everyone can improve their flexibility levels at any age, no matter what their starting flexibility levels are. It just takes a little bit of practice and consistency.

**When there's no pain, there's no gain.** Stretching should not be painful. Yes, you should feel a gentle pull on the muscle, but it should never be painful. Once you are in pain, your body will be tensing up, and you can't relax into a stretch if you are resisting in pain. If you are feeling pain, just back out of the stretch a bit. You may also not be ready for that particular stretch yet.

**If you are flexible. you don't need to stretch.** We all need to stretch, and the aging process does not exclude the flexible. The benefits of stretching go beyond flexibility alone. Generally, just because you are flexible in one area doesn't mean your entire body is flexible, so focus on your tighter areas.

**You should stretch before you work out or exercise.** Dynamic stretching can be done before a workout, but passive and static stretching should only be done after a workout. Stretching before you work out can decrease your lower body strength by more than 8 percent according to a study published in *The Journal of Strength and Conditioning Research*. This means static stretching before you exercise or play sports would decrease your performance levels.

**It's best to hold a stretch for 20 to 30 seconds.** Every fitness certification I have done tells people to hold a stretch for 10 to 30 seconds and repeat it two to four times. From my 18 years of experience, I can tell you that this is not effective. The longer you hold a stretch, the more benefits you will gain. A study published in *Sports Biomechanics* analyzed the amount of time it took to increase hip flexibility in a stretch. They found there was an increase after 1 minute, but there was a further increase at 5 minutes.

There are several myths that lead to some common stretching mistakes. I believe people fall for these myths because they tend to originate from a time before there was a lot of research, so they've been around for a while. These are five mistakes people often make when stretching:

**Pushing through pain.** That mindset of "No pain, no gain" has really become problematic. You do not want to be in pain when you stretch. If you are in pain, come out of the stretch and try it again with a smaller range of motion. If it still feels painful, you could see if there is a modification or prop you can use to make the stretch more comfortable.

**Not being consistent.** Stretching once a month is not going to make a big difference. You have to be consistent with your routine. I have seen clients make progress with just two stretching sessions a week, so you don't have to stretch every single day to make progress—you just have to be consistent each week.

**Creating more stress and tension.** Oftentimes I see people creating even more tension in their bodies when trying to stretch. This is not what you want! Make sure you check in with your jaw, neck, and shoulders during every stretch to make sure they are soft and relaxed.

**Stretching without warming up the body.** You will have a much more pleasant and effective stretching practice if your body is warmed up first. You could do this with dynamic stretching, a brisk walk, or any light exercise, or you could do it after a sauna or soak. Your body naturally warms up as the day goes on, so if you are someone who is super tight, you may want to practice your stretching later in the day.

**Not holding a stretch long enough.** As I have said before, it takes time for your body to relax into a stretch. Make sure you hold a stretch long enough to reach that point of softening when the stretch becomes more comfortable.

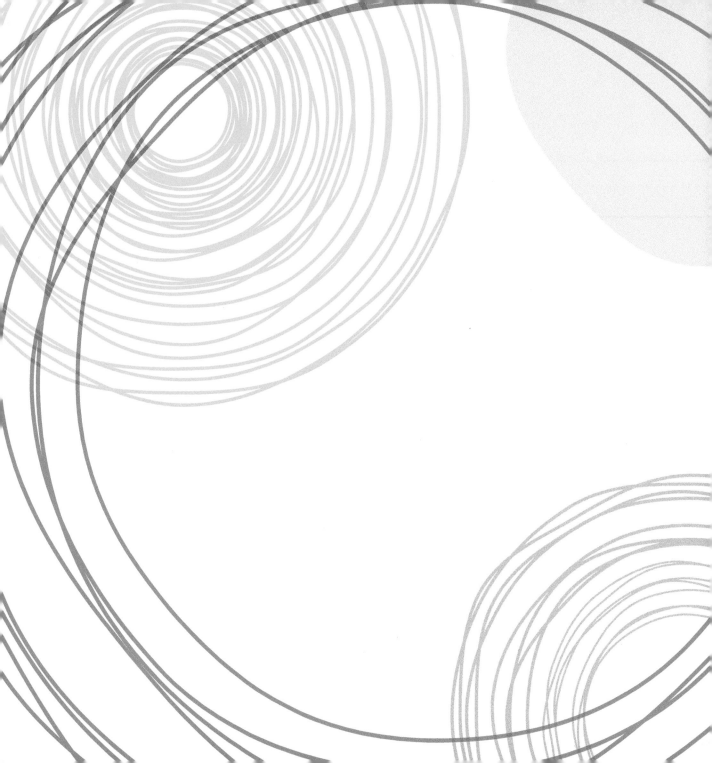

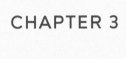

CHAPTER 3

# Making It a Regular Practice

You can use this book to create truly unique routines for all of your needs. Be sure to refer to the "Change It Up" feature that modifies each stretch in this book so you can find the best variation for your body. I recommend trying all of the individual stretches and making notes about which ones you feel your body needs the most. Then try looking through the routines to see which ones fit your lifestyle best. Don't forget to read chapter 16 to learn more about creating your own customized stretching routines.

# Everyone Is Different

I have never had two clients with the exact same issues, even if they've had the same injury. We are all unique, and we all have different expectations about how we want our body to feel and move. Even in our lifetime, our flexibility and expectations of it can change. It is important to be realistic about any limitations you have. Listen to your body and only do what feels comfortable and healthy.

# Stretching at Every Stage of Life

Stretching is wonderful for your body no matter what age you are. This is what you can expect of your muscles with each passing decade, and the common changes and ailments people in each age group experience.

## 20s

This is truly the prime of your life. Your flexibility and mobility should be at their best. If you are already tight at this age, it is important to start stretching now!

## 30s

In your thirties you will begin to lose muscle mass at a rate of 3 to 5 percent per decade, and your metabolism will start to decrease 2 to 3 percent each decade as well. Collagen and elastin levels also begin to decrease, which you may notice as fine lines in your skin, but the same thing is also happening inside your connective tissue.

## 40s

Your body starts to go through quite a few changes at this age. Metabolism slows down, muscle mass slowly decreases, and eyesight can change. Years of beating your body up may start catching up with you as you experience more aches and pains.

## 50s

Every decade after 40, we lose about a half inch of our height. Exercising regularly can prevent this. This is the decade your hormones change and it becomes harder to bounce back from illness and injuries.

## 60s

In your sixties you lose muscle mass at a much quicker rate than over the course of the last three decades. According to an article published by Harvard Health, men lose between 25 and 33 percent of their muscle mass in their sixties. Working out and stretching are highly important to prevent this.

## 70s

Certain medications and health ailments tend to be common among 70-year-olds. This can make falls much more likely, which means it is more important than ever at this age to work on your balance, strength, and flexibility.

## 80s

Mobility, strength, and balance can greatly decrease by this point, which can lead to issues with walking and caring for yourself. We do still have the potential to build muscle mass in our eighties, so even if you are in this age group, you can improve!

## 90s

Stamina and strength are decreasing, making it more difficult to take care of yourself. In a study of 5,900 individuals in their nineties, 75 percent of women and 59 percent of men reported struggling to walk half a mile. This doesn't have to be the case if you keep up with stretching and exercise.

As you can see, it is incredibly important to take care of our bodies well throughout the decades! You will only lose muscle mass, balance, and mobility if you don't work on preserving them.

# Consider Your Options

In my opinion, the most difficult part of stretching is making it part of your daily routine. The challenge is simply creating a new habit. If you are going to implement a stretching routine, then maybe you would like to add breathing, meditation, or journaling as part of the routine too. I strongly encourage you to incorporate other self-care practices into your stretching. You may want to start a breathing or meditation practice to begin or end your sessions. The whole point of the physical practice of yoga is to prepare the body and mind to sit still in meditation. If you could fit in 5 minutes of breathing, 10 minutes of stretching, and 5 minutes of meditation, then you would have a 20-minute routine that would be beneficial on a wide variety of levels.

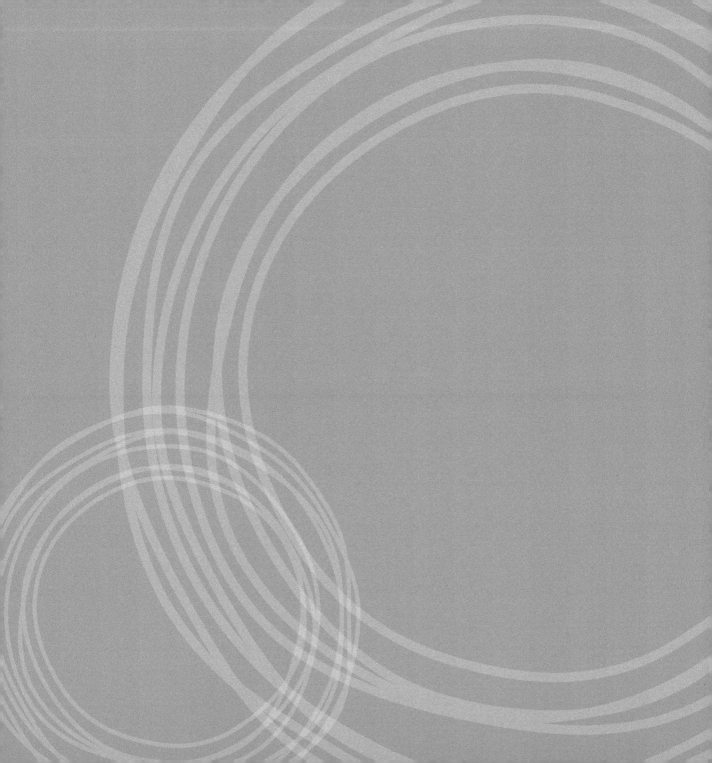

"Training for strength and flexibility is a must. You must use it to support your techniques. Techniques alone are no good if you don't support them with strength and flexibility."

—BRUCE LEE

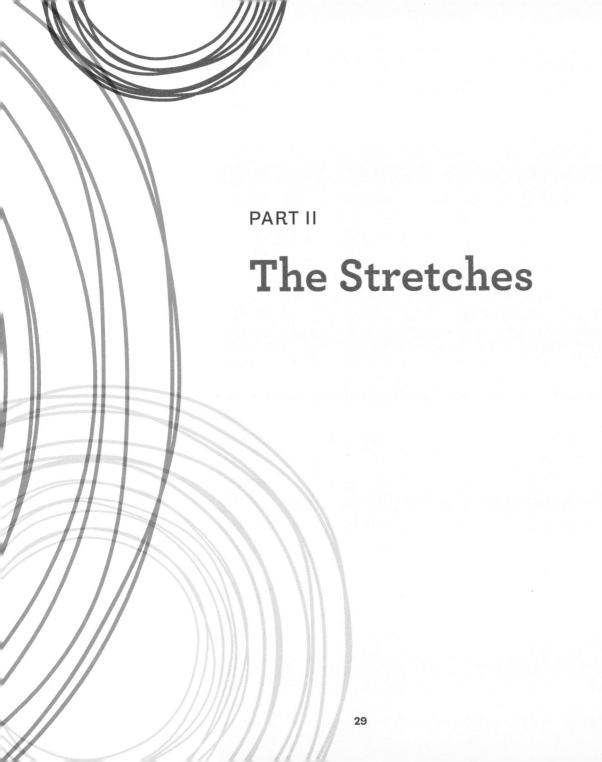

PART II

# The Stretches

# HOW TO USE THE STRETCHES

Now that we have covered the fundamentals of stretching, it is time to learn the 60 essential stretches that your body needs in order to stay fit and healthy for a lifetime! In this section you will learn simple stretches that you can do to target each part of your body. Each chapter is organized by muscle group so you can work through the stretches one problem area at a time if you would like.

The best way to approach these individual stretches is by taking the time to look at the illustration, read the numbered instructions, and go over the tips and modifications on how to change it up. Then go ahead and try out that stretch in your own body. If you feel any pain or major restrictions, you should stop and try the modified version. If you are not feeling like you got a good stretch, try the advanced variation. Take the time to be mindful and notice what muscles you are feeling the stretch in. As you move through the stretches, you will become highly aware of which ones your body needs the most.

Part III will group these stretches together in focused 10-minute routines, which is easy for anyone to find the time for! Remember, it doesn't take a big time commitment to improve your flexibility. Being consistent with short, 10-minute routines is all that you need to see improvement. You will be amazed at how quickly you start feeling and moving better.

# MUSCLES OF THE HUMAN BODY

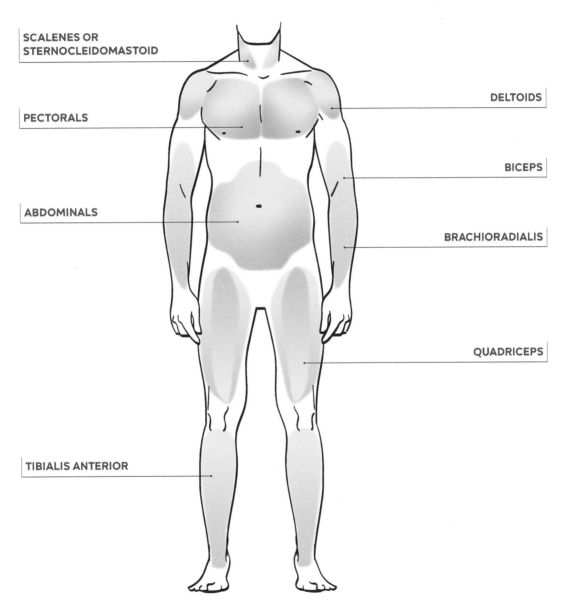

SCALENES OR
STERNOCLEIDOMASTOID

PECTORALS

ABDOMINALS

TIBIALIS ANTERIOR

DELTOIDS

BICEPS

BRACHIORADIALIS

QUADRICEPS

# MUSCLES OF THE HUMAN BODY

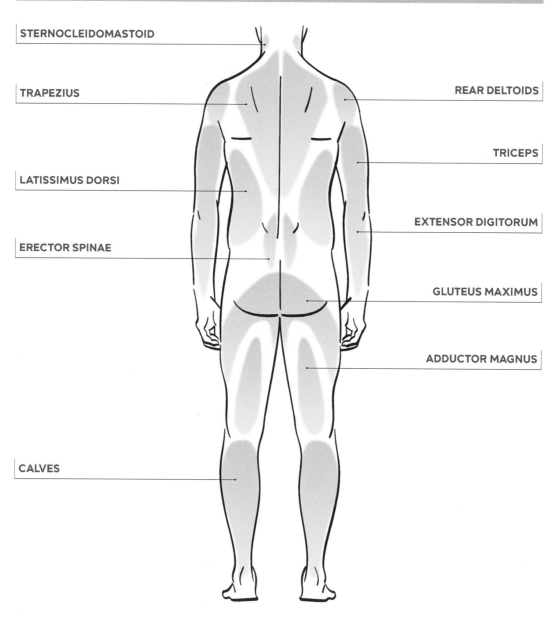

STERNOCLEIDOMASTOID

TRAPEZIUS

LATISSIMUS DORSI

ERECTOR SPINAE

CALVES

REAR DELTOIDS

TRICEPS

EXTENSOR DIGITORUM

GLUTEUS MAXIMUS

ADDUCTOR MAGNUS

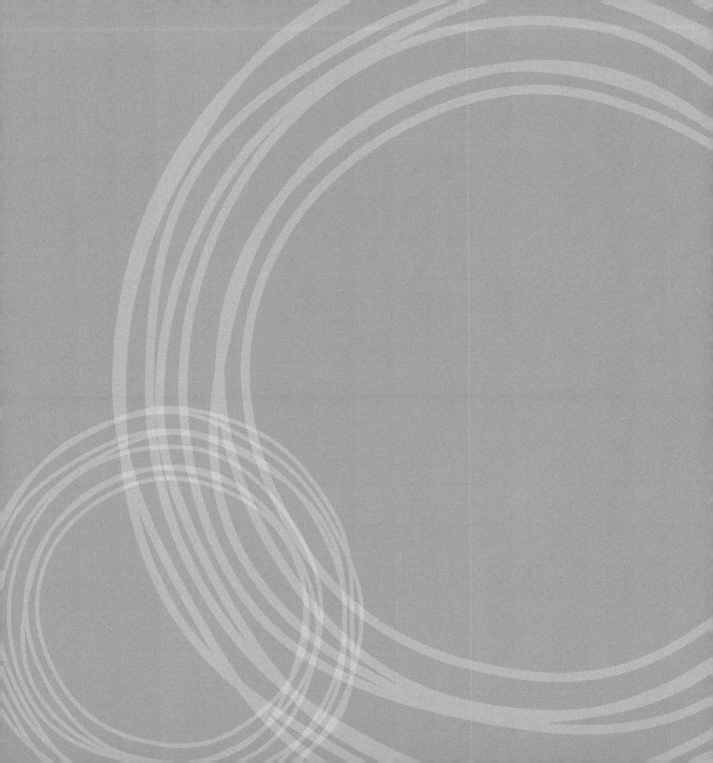

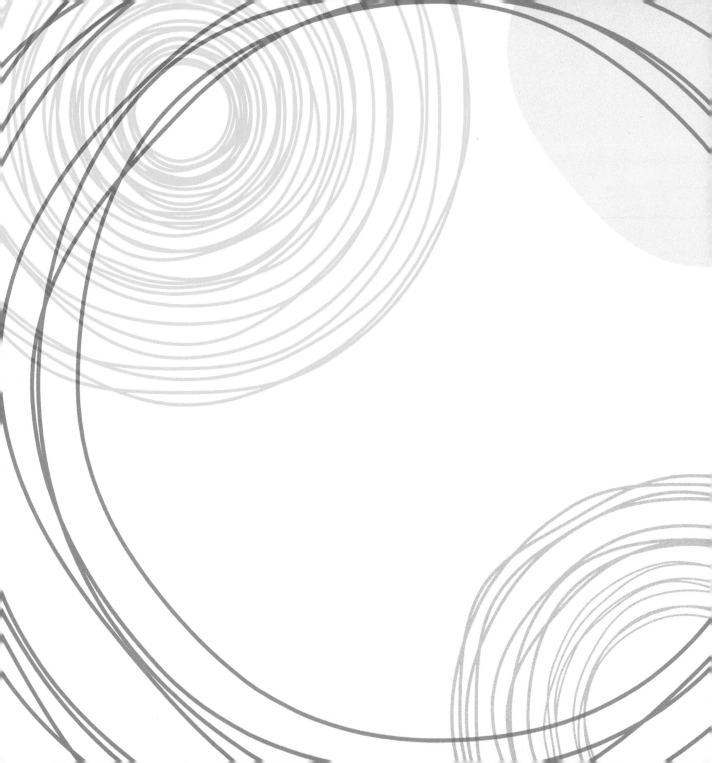

CHAPTER 4

# Neck

# HEAD TURNS

## Type of Stretch

- Dynamic stretch
- Static stretch

## Main Motion(s)

- Rotation

## Affected Area(s)

- Neck, scalenes, trapezius

## Good For

- This stretch can prevent the loss of neck mobility as you age, which can interfere with your ability to drive and other daily activities. This stretch also reduces tension in your neck.

## Instructions

1. Sit in a chair and use good posture.
2. Slowly turn your head to the right as far as you can.
3. Hold your neck in this position for 10 seconds.
4. Slowly turn your head to the left as far as you can.
5. Hold your neck in this position for 10 seconds.
6. Repeat 5 times to the right and to the left.

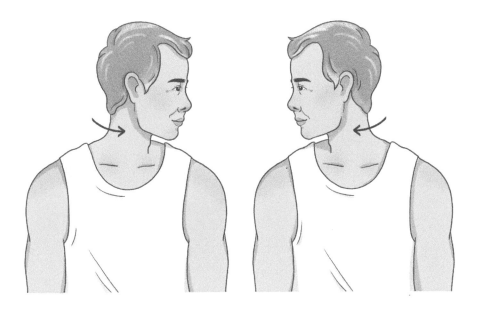

## Change It Up

- Take your time and move slowly. You can make this a dynamic stretch by continually turning your head left and right with a small pause on each side. You can also use this as a static stretch by holding your head turned to the side for a longer amount of time.
- You can make this stretch into a small balance challenge by doing it standing up. The closer you place your feet together, the harder it is to balance.

## Remember

- Sit up tall while keeping your shoulders down and relaxed to get the most out of this stretch.

# HEAD NODS

## Type of Stretch

- Dynamic stretch
- Static stretch

## Main Motion(s)

- Flexion, extension

## Affected Area(s)

- Neck

## Good For

- This helps increase neck flexibility and can improve forward head posture. It is an excellent physical therapy exercise for whiplash and neck pain.

## Instructions

1. Sit up tall and inhale as you slowly lift your chin toward the sky. Go slowly until you feel a nice stretch in the front of your neck.

2. Return your head to the starting position.

3. Exhale as you pull your chin down to your chest and pause.

4. Repeat 10 times.

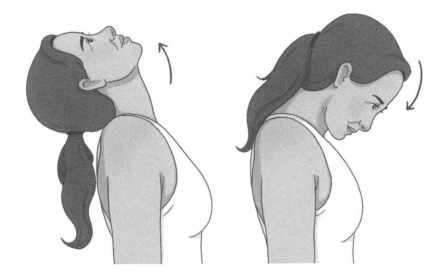

## Change It Up

- Neck muscles are small and delicate, making them easier to pull. Make sure you move slowly from one position to the other. If you want to make it a static stretch, hold the stretch for a longer period instead of just pausing at your end range.
- Try doing this dynamic stretch standing up with your feet together and eyes closed to challenge your balance too. You could also do it in an all-fours position to see how gravity changes the stretch.

## Remember

- If you feel any discomfort as you tilt your head back, come back to neutral and try retracting your chin back slightly before you try again.

# EAR TO SHOULDER

## Type of Stretch

- Static stretch

## Main Motion(s)

- Lateral flexion

## Affected Area(s)

- Neck, scalenes, trapezius

## Good For

- The three sets of scalene muscles not only cause pain when they are tight, but they also restrict your neck from moving in its full range of motion. This stretch will help reduce tension and pain in the neck and shoulders.

## Instructions

1. Sit up tall with a long spine.
2. Bring your right hand down by your side and reach strongly through the fingertips.
3. Place your left hand on top of your head and gently pull your neck toward your left shoulder.
4. Hold for 30 seconds or more.
5. Switch sides.

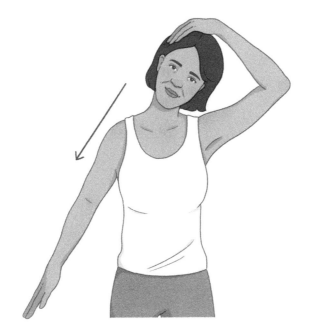

## Change It Up

- If your neck is feeling tender, it is best not to add the weight of your hand on your head. In this case, you can interlace your hands behind your back and gently reach downward while bringing your ear to your shoulder.
- Instead of reaching straight down, you can bend your elbow and place your hand as far behind your back as you can.

## Remember

- Actively reaching through your fingertips changes the stretch. Make sure you aren't just letting the arm hang loosely.

# HALF CIRCLES

## Type of Stretch

- Dynamic stretch

## Main Motion(s)

- Rotation

## Affected Area(s)

- Neck, scalenes, trapezius

## Good For

- This stretch is great for opening up the neck muscles at almost every angle. It is a great way to relieve stress and tension from the neck and shoulders.

## Instructions

1. Sit up tall with a straight spine.

2. Start by bringing your ear toward your right shoulder.

3. Slowly begin to rotate your head forward in a half circle.

4. Once your ear is over your left shoulder, slowly rotate your head back to your right shoulder.

5. Continue to repeat half circles 5 to 10 times.

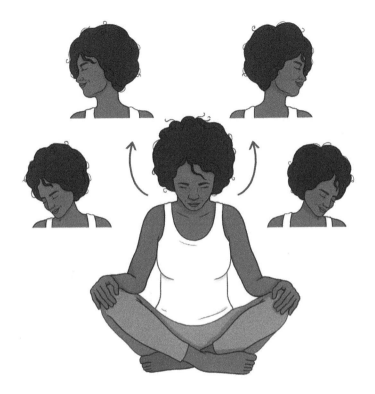

## Change It Up

- If your neck is feeling tender, try doing quarter circles. You can just move your head from the ear-to-shoulder position to the chin-to-chest position.
- You can make this stretch more intense by reaching your arms behind you, interlacing your fingers together, and pulling down toward the floor.

## Remember

- Make sure you don't get tempted to do a full circle. Research has shown that moving the head backward while rotating the neck can place unnecessary stress on the cervical spine.

# NECK RETRACTIONS

## Type of Stretch

- Active stretch
- Dynamic stretch

## Main Motion(s)

- Retraction

## Affected Area(s)

- Neck

## Good For

- This is the best stretching exercise for reversing forward head posture and rounded shoulders. It can be very helpful for people who suffer from headaches, neck pain, shoulder pain, or upper back tension.

## Instructions

1. Sit up tall with a straight spine.
2. Pull your chin and head straight backward.
3. Return to neutral position and repeat 20 times.

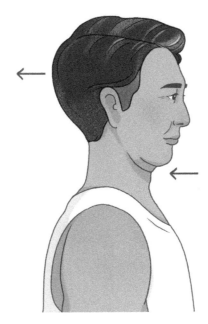

## Change It Up

- Try doing this seated or standing in front of a wall. It is nice to have the tactile sensation of the wall behind you to give you a goal of how far to retract.
- Try holding the retraction phase longer for a challenging active stretch that will help strengthen your neck muscles too.

## Remember

- This is a great exercise to do while driving. We tend to have forward head posture while driving, and the driver's seat is a great place to work on fixing it. First make sure your headrest isn't encouraging forward head posture, and then you can do this exercise using the headrest as the goal for how far back to retract.

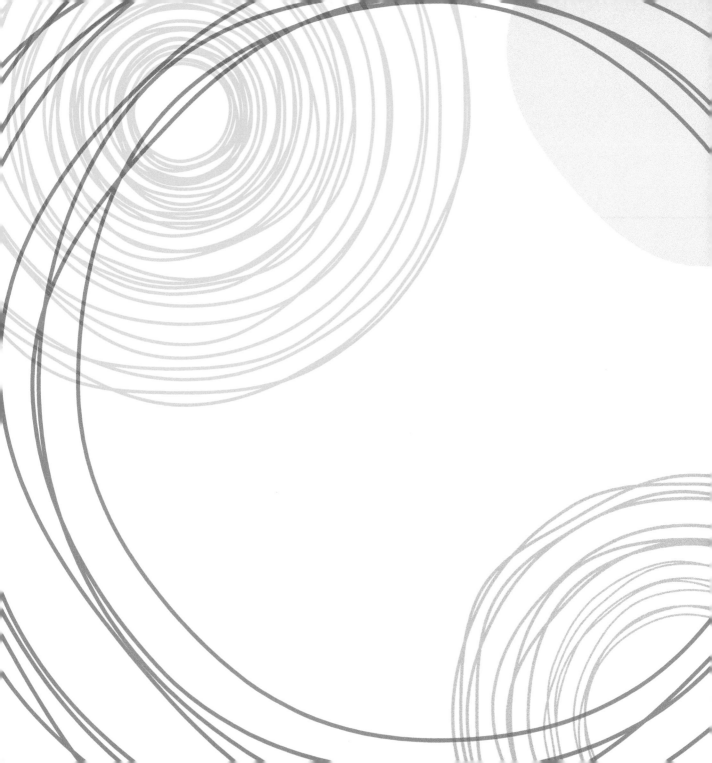

CHAPTER 5

# Arms and Shoulders

# SHOULDER SHRUG AND RELEASE

## Type of Stretch
- Dynamic stretch

## Main Motion(s)
- Elevation, depression

## Affected Area(s)
- Shoulders, trapezius

## Good For
- Actively contracting the trapezius muscles and quickly relaxing them will help decrease the tension in all the surrounding neck and shoulder muscles. This stretch can be wonderful for stress relief and is a perfect break you can take right at your desk.

## Instructions

1. Sitting up tall, inhale as you shrug your shoulders up to your ears and create more tension in the neck and shoulders for a brief second.

2. Exhale and quickly let your shoulders drop down to the starting position.

3. Repeat 5 to 10 times.

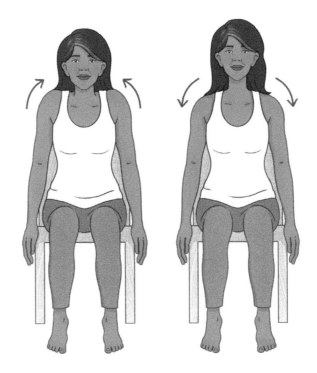

## Change It Up

- Make sure you sit up tall with your shoulders pulled back slightly so you are in good alignment. Don't overlook syncing your breath with the movement. Exhaling as you release the tension will help your body relax on a much deeper level.
- Try squeezing the muscles for a full 10 seconds at the top of the motion and you will isometrically strengthen the trapezius muscle before you stretch it.

## Remember

- Do this stretch seated. You will have a much greater release of tension if your entire body can relax.

# SHOULDER CIRCLES

**Type of Stretch**

- Dynamic stretch

**Main Motion(s)**

- Rotation

**Affected Area(s)**

- Shoulders

**Good For**

- This is a great warm-up for any upper body activity or racquet sport. It will help improve your range of motion in the shoulder joint and can also help improve posture.

**Instructions**

1. Stand with your feet about hip width apart.

2. Reach your arms straight up above you.

3. Start to bring your arms down in front of you in the largest circle you can.

4. Continue making circles 5 to 10 times or more.

5. Then repeat in a backward circle.

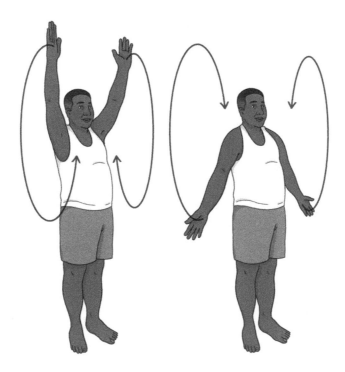

## Change It Up

- If you have any shoulder issues, you may want to do this stretch one arm at a time. Take a much slower approach and try to gently explore how big of a circle you can make.
- If you would like to work on coordination, try moving one arm forward while the other arm moves in backward circles. The closer together your feet are, the more challenging balance becomes.

## Remember

- Do this while standing up tall with your core engaged. You can move quickly to warm up the shoulder and slowly to truly find the full range of motion.

# CROSS BODY STRETCH

## Type of Stretch

- Dynamic stretch
- Static stretch

## Main Motion(s)

- Abduction

## Affected Area(s)

- Shoulders

## Good For

- This motion helps stretch and decrease tension in the posterior shoulder muscles. Many people enjoy using this as a dynamic stretch in between weight lifting exercises.

## Instructions

1. Bring your right arm across your body and use your left arm to support it by grabbing near the elbow.

2. Gently pull the arm across until you feel a nice stretch in the shoulder.

3. Hold for 1 minute and repeat on the other arm.

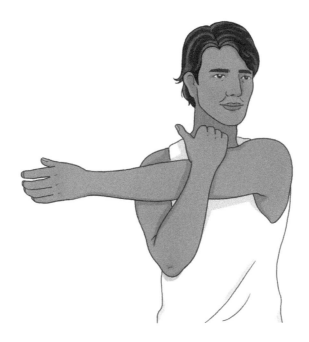

## Change It Up

- If you want to do this as a dynamic stretch, you will only hold for about 5 seconds before switching sides. You can alternate a few times back and forth. This can make it a great break between exercises.
- You can try retracting the shoulder blade before you pull your arm across to intensify the stretch. Try to keep the shoulder blade retracted throughout the movement and stretch.

## Remember

- For better alignment, once you reach your arm straight out, soften and relax your shoulder down before you pull it across. Take slow deep breaths to help your body relax.

# OVERHEAD TRICEP

## Type of Stretch

- Static stretch

## Main Motion(s)

- Flexion

## Affected Area(s)

- Triceps, shoulders

## Good For

- This stretch helps open up the shoulder joint and stretches the triceps muscles. It is a great stretch to do after upper body activities like racquet sports.

## Instructions

1. Bring your right arm overhead and bend the right elbow.

2. Place your left hand on top of the right elbow.

3. Gently guide your elbow toward your head and farther back.

4. Take slow deep breaths and switch sides after 1 minute.

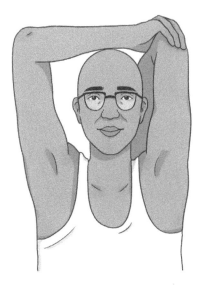
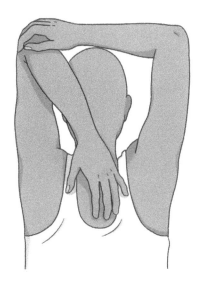

### Change It Up

- You can use a strap to make this stretch more comfortable. Place the strap in the hand you are reaching overhead with and bend your elbow. Reach the opposite hand behind your back to give the strap a pull downward to assist you deeper into the stretch.
- If you feel any numbness or tingling in your arm, hand, or fingers, you may want to come out of the stretch and try again.

### Remember

- Make sure your body doesn't try to overcompensate for this movement. If you feel your rib cage open wide or your back arch, back out of the stretch slightly.

# FOLD WITH HANDS INTERLACED

## Type of Stretch

- Static stretch

## Main Motion(s)

- Hyperextension

## Affected Area(s)

- Shoulders, chest, hamstrings

## Good For

- This stretch is a great way to open up the chest and shoulders. It also helps improve posture and increase shoulder mobility.

## Instructions

1. Stand with your feet wide apart and toes turned slightly outward.

2. Interlace your hands behind your back and start to lift them as high as you can.

3. Fold forward and bring your arms with you, trying to reach overhead toward the floor.

4. Take slow deep breaths while you try to elongate your spine.

5. When you are ready to stand back up, you can release your hands to make it easier.

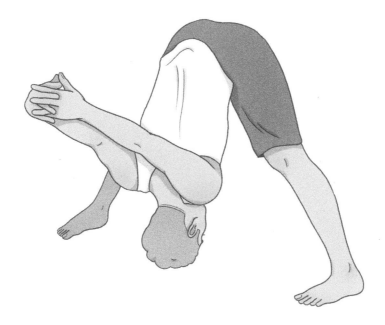

## Change It Up

- One way to modify this stretch is by holding a strap instead of interlacing your hands. This will allow your arms to be wider apart so they can move farther.
- Placing your feet together will make this stretch more challenging in terms of balance and hamstring flexibility.

## Remember

- Try to keep your arms and legs straight to get the most out of this stretch.
- Contraindications: pregnancy, uncontrolled high blood pressure, sinusitis, and glaucoma.

# BACK SCRATCH

## Type of Stretch

- Static stretch

## Main Motion(s)

- Internal and external shoulder rotation

## Affected Area(s)

- Shoulders, triceps

## Good For

- This stretch helps eliminate rounded shoulders and releases tension in the chest, shoulders, and triceps.

## Instructions

1. Reach your right arm straight up to the sky and bend your right elbow.

2. Walk your right fingertips down your spine as far as you can.

3. Reach your left arm behind your back and bend your left elbow to reach upward.

4. Walk your left fingertips up your spine as much as you can.

5. Try to touch or interlace your fingers and hold for 1 minute.

6. Repeat on the other side.

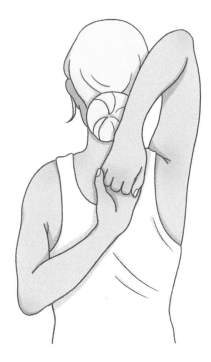

## Change It Up

- You can place a hand towel, strap, or belt in your top hand and let it hang behind your back. Reach your other hand behind you to grab the towel and walk your hand up it as much as you can. This will help you hold the stretch better if your hands can't touch.
- Lift the top elbow straight up toward the ceiling to help intensify the stretch.

## Remember

- This position can make you curl forward, so try sitting up tall to improve your alignment and posture.

# ARM SWINGS

## Type of Stretch

- Dynamic stretch

## Main Motion(s)

- Abduction, adduction

## Affected Area(s)

- Shoulders, arms

## Good For

- This is a great stretch to warm up the arms and shoulders for any activity. It quickly increases blood flow and improves mobility.

## Instructions

1. Stand with your feet wide apart.

2. Bring your arms out wide and start to swing them to cross in front of your body.

3. Let them swing open as wide as you can.

4. Keep swinging your arms back and forth, alternating which arm is on top.

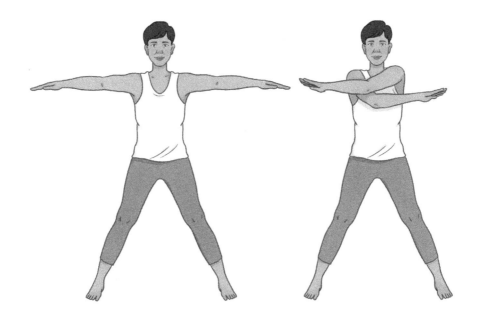

## Change It Up

- If it doesn't feel good to swing your arms, you can take this much slower and simply hold your arms crossed in front of you in each position and then open your arms out wide. This would turn it into a static stretch, so it wouldn't be recommended as a warm-up.
- It feels really nice to add a twisting movement from side to side as you swing your arms back and forth.

## Remember

- Standing with your feet wide apart gives you a more stable base in regard to balance. It's better to have your feet wide in this exercise so you can move freely without worrying about balance.

# CLASPED ARM EXTENSION

## Type of Stretch

- Static stretch

## Main Motion(s)

- Flexion

## Affected Area(s)

- Shoulders, lower neck, upper back

## Good For

- This stretch helps improve your posture and reduce tension. It is wonderful for rowers or anyone with a lot of tension in between the shoulder blades. This can happen from upper body workouts or squeezing the upper back muscles to encourage good posture.

## Instructions

1. Stand up tall and interlace your hands together in front of you.

2. Reach your arms straight out as far as you can.

3. Broaden your shoulder blades wide apart while you push through the hands.

4. Pull your chin down toward your chest.

5. Hold for 15 seconds, release, and repeat 1 to 3 more times.

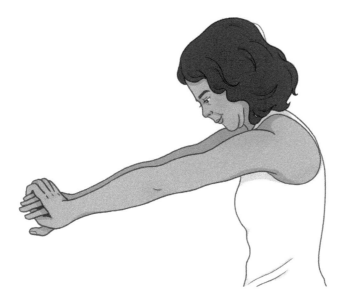

## Change It Up

- You do not have to pull your chin to your chest. If you are experiencing any neck problems by pulling your chin down, leave your head in a neutral position to only focus on the upper back and shoulders..
- Visualize your shoulder blades sliding farther apart from each other as you reach strongly through your hands.

## Remember

- Make sure you do not lean forward in this stretch. Focus on standing up tall and creating space between the shoulder blades instead.

# THREAD THE NEEDLE

## Type of Stretch

- Static stretch

## Main Motion(s)

- Hip, knee, and ankle flexion; horizontal shoulder adduction

## Affected Area(s)

- Shoulders, neck, back

## Good For

- This stretch can help you calm down and release stress. It helps open up your chest, neck, and shoulders while lengthening your spine.

## Instructions

1. Come down onto your hands and knees in an all-fours position.

2. Reach your right arm under your left arm as far as you can.

3. Place your right shoulder and ear down onto the floor.

4. Extend your left arm out straight.

5. Release after 1 minute and repeat on the other side.

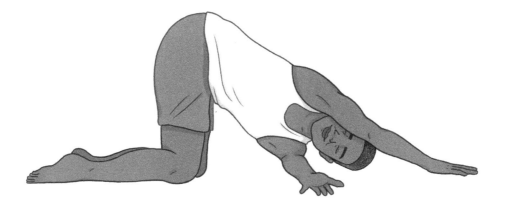

## Change It Up

- You can use props to make this more comfortable. Try using a folded blanket under your knees to provide a cushion, or under your head if it doesn't quite reach the floor.
- If your head is resting on the floor, you can take your straight arm and bend it, reaching behind your lower back, to help deepen the twist.

## Remember

- Try to keep your hips directly above your knees for the entire stretch. It can be helpful to walk your fingers as far over as you can before bringing your shoulder down to the floor.
- Contraindications: knee, neck, or shoulder injuries.

# STIR THE POT

### Type of Stretch
- Dynamic stretch

### Main Motion(s)
- Rotation

### Affected Area(s)
- Shoulders, arms

### Good For
- This stretch helps improve circulation in the arm, making it great to do before you work out or in between exercises to help your muscles recover. It can also be very beneficial for frozen shoulder and other shoulder injuries.

### Instructions

1. Stand in a lunge position and place your hand on your front leg or table for support.

2. Keep your spine long and core engaged.

3. Let your other arm hang down loose and make 20 clockwise circles with your arm.

4. Switch to 20 counterclockwise circles.

5. Switch arms and repeat.

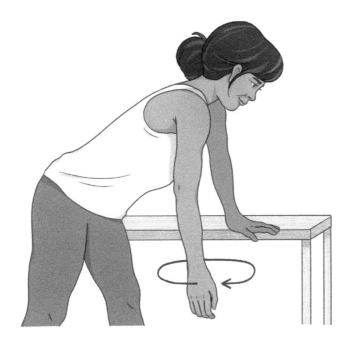

## Change It Up

- If you have lower back issues, it can be more ideal to place your hand on a table or chair for support so you can bend over to the angle that feels comfortable to you.
- You could add a small dumbbell (one to three pounds) to help the hand get heavy and stretch further. You could also just use visualization to help think about your arm becoming as long as possible while doing the rotations.

## Remember

- Watch out for tension in the neck and shoulders to make sure you are not placing too much pressure on your supporting arm.

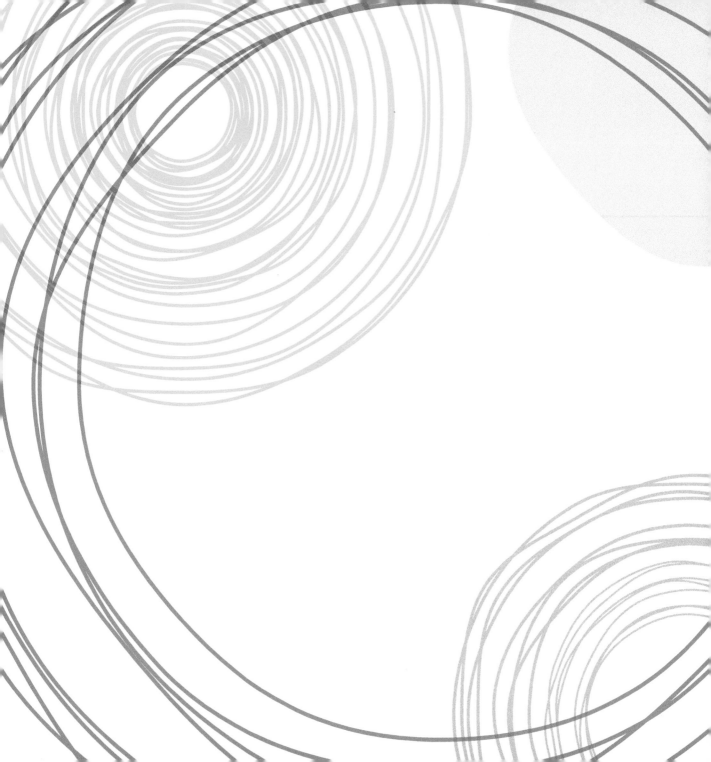

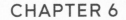

CHAPTER 6

# Wrists and Hands

# WRIST ROLL OUT

## Type of Stretch

- Dynamic stretch

## Main Motion(s)

- Rotation

## Affected Area(s)

- Wrists, forearms, hands

## Good For

- This stretch helps lubricate the wrist joint, making it ideal therapy for carpal tunnel syndrome and arthritis. It can also be helpful after doing push-ups, planks, or any other activity that has you down on your hands.

## Instructions

1. Hold your arm at a 90-degree angle.

2. Keep your hand flat with fingers together and begin making 15 to 20 clockwise circular movements.

3. Repeat 15 to 20 times in the opposite direction.

4. Switch hands.

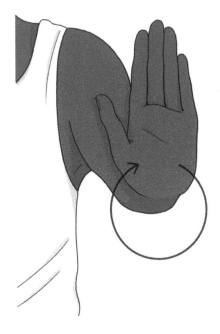

## Change It Up

- You can make a soft fist instead of a flat hand for a gentler stretch. If you have severe arthritis, this may be a better variation for you.
- Try doing the same movement with a soft fist and notice which variation you prefer.

## Remember

- Moving quickly can be great for warming up the wrist, but moving slowly will allow you to move in your absolute full range of motion. Notice at which angles your wrist doesn't move as smoothly and focus on that part of the circle.

# WRIST FLEXION

## Type of Stretch

- Static stretch

## Main Motion(s)

- Flexion

## Affected Area(s)

- Wrists, forearms, hands

## Good For

- This is a great warm-up for the wrists, and it reverses being in push-up or plank position, so it can be a nice stretch after an upper body workout.

## Instructions

1. Come down onto your hands and knees in an all-fours position.

2. Place your hands in front of you with the tops facing down.

3. Slowly begin to sit back toward your heels.

4. Hold for 1 minute.

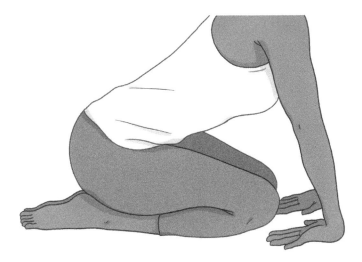

## Change It Up

- This stretch can be very intense. If it feels like too much on your wrists, you can do a gentler version seated or standing. Extend your arms in front of you and use one hand to stretch the other by pulling your fingers downward with your palm facing down.
- The further you sit back toward your heels, the more intense the stretch becomes. If it still doesn't feel like the stretch you need, move your hands further in front of you and sit back toward your heels again.

## Remember

- Pay attention to the rest of your body too! Make sure you are not sitting awkwardly or creating more tension in your body.

# WRIST EXTENSION

## Type of Stretch

- Static stretch

## Main Motion(s)

- Extension

## Affected Area(s)

- Wrists, forearms

## Good For

- This motion helps stretch the wrists and forearms. It can be helpful therapy for carpal tunnel syndrome and wrist injuries. It is also an excellent cooldown stretch for athletes who wrestle, box, play racquet sports, or golf.

## Instructions

1. Come down onto your hands and knees in an all-fours position.

2. Place your palms on the floor and turn your fingertips to point toward you.

3. Slowly sit back toward your heels.

4. Hold for 1 minute.

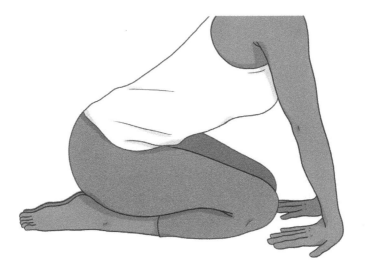

### Change It Up

- You can place your hands closer to your knees if you need to decrease the intensity of the stretch. Make sure you keep your arms straight. If it still feels too intense, try doing this stretch while standing with your hands on a table.
- The further your hands are in front of you, the more challenging the stretch becomes as you sit back toward your heels.

### Remember

- Pay attention to your neck and shoulders to make sure they are relaxed. Try to keep your head and neck aligned with the rest of your spine.

# HANDS AND KNEES WRIST CIRCLES

### Type of Stretch

- Dynamic stretch

### Main Motion(s)

- Rotation

### Affected Area(s)

- Wrists, forearms

### Good For

- This stretch helps warm up the wrists at every angle possible, and the circular movement is also beneficial for arthritis. It is a wonderful way to prepare for upper body activities.

### Instructions

1. Come down onto your hands and knees in an all-fours position.

2. Place your hands on the floor with your palms down and fingers pointed outward.

3. Begin to move your body in a circular motion, alternating clockwise and counterclockwise for 10 to 20 circles in each direction.

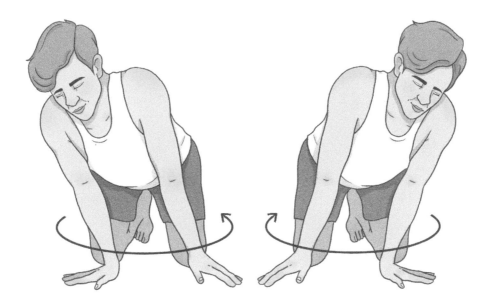

## Change It Up

- If it is difficult for you to be on your hands and knees, try this stretch while standing with your hands on a table or slightly below shoulder level on a wall in front of you.
- Keep your arms straight to get the most out of this stretch. Start off with small circles and slowly let them begin to get larger.

## Remember

- Be curious about how tiny of a circle you can make and how big your circles can be. Different movements will help different muscles in the wrists, forearms, and shoulders get more out of the stretch.

# FINGER SPREAD

## Type of Stretch

- Dynamic stretch

## Main Motion(s)

- Abduction

## Affected Area(s)

- Hands, fingers

## Good For

- This motion helps stretch all the muscles in your hands and fingers. This is a great stretch for artists, laborers, gardeners, writers, typists, or anyone who uses their hands a lot.

## Instructions

1. Hold out your right palm in a straight position with your fingers squeezed together.

2. Spread your fingers apart as wide as possible and let your palm stretch open.

3. Bring your fingers back together and repeat 10 times.

4. Switch hands.

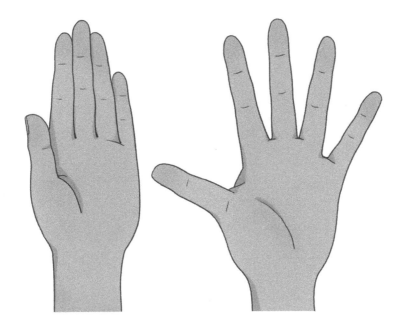

## Change It Up

- If you have arthritis, try doing this very slowly and gently. Hold the stretch for as long as you can and repeat until you have held the stretch for a full minute.
- You can place a rubber band around your fingers and thumb to provide extra resistance to stretch against. This will help you both strengthen and stretch the fingers.

## Remember

- Although you could do both hands at the same time, you will get more out of the stretch by giving your full attention to one hand at a time.

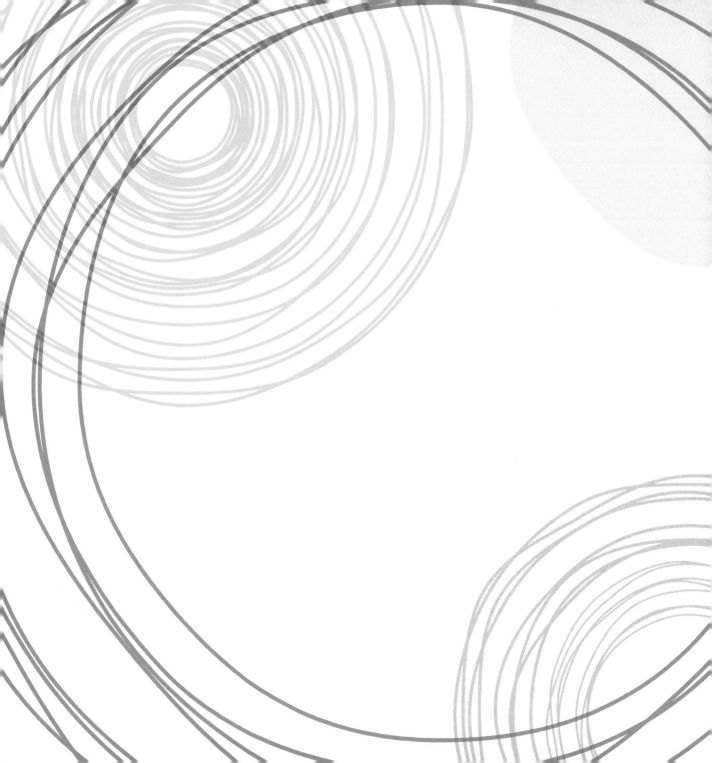

CHAPTER 7

# Torso and Back

# SEATED CAT COW

## Type of Stretch

- Dynamic stretch

## Main Motion(s)

- Flexion, extension

## Affected Area(s)

- Neck, back, shoulders, torso

## Good For

- This stretch helps open up the spine and can decrease tension and reduce pain in the neck, shoulders, and lower back. It's a great midday break at the office.

## Instructions

1. Sit down in a chair.

2. Place your hands on your knees.

3. Exhale as you round your spine while curling your chin to your chest and tucking your hips and tailbone under.

4. Come back to your starting position.

5. Inhale as you sit up as tall as you can and push your heart and rib cage forward as you lift your chin.

6. Continue to flow from one position to the other 10 times.

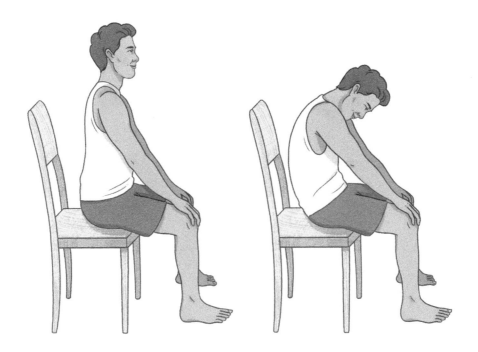

## Change It Up

- Take your time and be mindful to move every part of your spine into the fullest stretch.
- Close your eyes and visualize creating more space in between each vertebra. Try to truly connect with your spine and notice where you are feeling the stretch.

## Remember

- Instead of pushing the chest forward to arch your back, try creating length in your torso and lifting your chest up toward the sky as you arch back.

# QUADRUPED CAT COW

## Type of Stretch

- Dynamic stretch

## Main Motion(s)

- Flexion, extension

## Affected Area(s)

- Back

## Good For

- This stretch helps decompress the spine and create more space between the vertebrae. It will improve the mobility of your spine, which is important for every single daily activity.

## Instructions

1. Come down onto your hands and knees in an all-fours position.

2. Round your back and imagine bringing your chin to your tailbone.

3. Return to a flat back.

4. Arch your back and let your rib cage become heavy. Imagine bringing the back of your head to your tailbone.

5. Continue to move back and forth between positions for 10 repetitions.

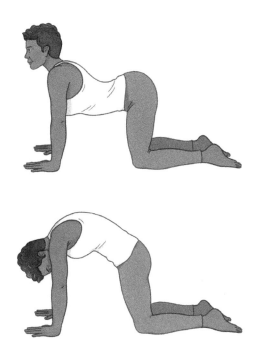

## Change It Up

- You can place your hands on yoga blocks or hold on to dumbbells to take pressure off your wrists.
- Tap into your curiosity. Play with small movements in your hips and shoulders by moving them side to side to create different stretches as you round and arch your back.

## Remember

- Take your time. You have to slow down and be mindful to get the most out of this stretch. Really pay attention to how much space you can create between each vertebra as you round your back.

# CHILD'S POSE

## Type of Stretch

- Static stretch

## Main Motion(s)

- Hip, knee, and back flexion

## Affected Area(s)

- Back, shoulders

## Good For

- This stretch helps decompress the lower back and is very restorative. Fifteen minutes in this position is equivalent to four hours of sleep.

## Instructions

1. Come down to a kneeling position and sit back toward your heels.

2. Spread your knees apart slightly wider than hip distance.

3. Walk your hands forward to rest your torso on your lap.

4. Bring your forehead to the ground.

5. Hold for at least 1 minute.

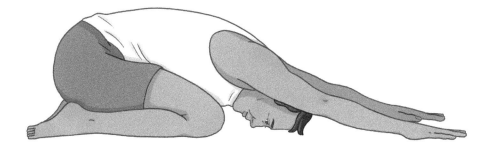

## Change It Up

- If your forehead cannot reach the ground, you can stack your fists on top of each other and rest your forehead on your fists, or grab a yoga block instead. You can also make this stretch more restorative by bringing your arms to your sides and reaching for your feet with your hands.
- You can bring your knees together to make the stretch slightly more challenging. Play with different knee positions to find the width that is ideal for you.

## Remember

- Connect to your breath and feel your belly expand against your thighs as you inhale, and let your spine sink down and soften as you exhale.
- If you're pregnant, use wide knees to avoid injury.

# SEATED TWIST

## Type of Stretch

- Static stretch

## Main Motion(s)

- Twisting

## Affected Area(s)

- Back, shoulders, chest, neck

## Good For

- This is an easy twist to help unravel tension and detoxify the organs. It is a great stretch for golfers and athletes in racquet sports to help increase their twisting mobility. The farther you can twist, the more power you will bring to your game.

## Instructions

1. Sit down in a cross-legged position.
2. Reach your left hand over to grab your right knee.
3. Place your right hand on the floor behind your back.
4. Sit up as tall as you can before you twist.
5. Turn your head and gaze to look over your shoulder.
6. Hold for 1 minute before you switch sides.

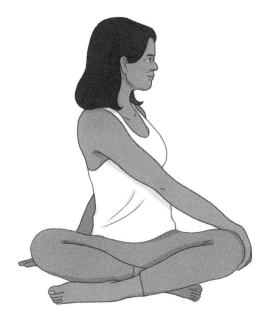

## Change It Up

- If it is uncomfortable to sit cross-legged, you can also do this stretch sitting in a chair.
- As you turn your head as far as you can, turn your gaze as far as you can too. This will help you deepen the twist.

## Remember

- You can't twist a rounded spine very well. Make sure you are sitting up tall, and think about creating length in your spine as you twist.

# SPHINX

## Type of Stretch

- Static stretch

## Main Motion(s)

- Extension

## Affected Area(s)

- Back, chest, shoulders

## Good For

- This is a gentle backbend that will help lengthen the torso and spine while stimulating digestion. This stretch can be therapeutic for herniated and bulging discs.

## Instructions

1. Lie down on your stomach with your hands under your shoulders.

2. Slide your elbows back so they align under your shoulders with your forearms parallel.

3. Lift your chin, chest, and torso up as much as you can.

4. Hold for 1 minute.

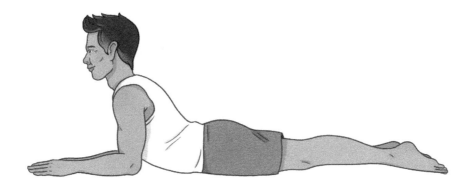

## Change It Up

- This is one of the gentlest backbends. You can spread your legs wider to help release tension in the sacrum. If even this feels too intense for you, try simply lying on your stomach. That alone may be a big enough stretch for you right now.
- Use a pillow or bolster under your forearms or straighten your arms to help deepen the stretch.

## Remember

- Instead of focusing on the backbend, try to think about creating length from your pubic bone to your ribs, from your ribs to your collarbones, and from your collarbones to your chin. Creating length in the front of your body will naturally bend the back side and keep you safe from injury.
- Contraindications: back injury, headache, and pregnancy.

# COBRA

## Type of Stretch

- Active stretch
- Static stretch

## Main Motion(s)

- Back extension

## Affected Area(s)

- Back, chest, shoulders

## Good For

- This is a moderate backbend that will help lengthen the spine and the abdomen. It can help soothe sciatica and lower back issues while stimulating digestion and being therapeutic for asthma.

## Instructions

1. Lie down on your stomach with your legs together.

2. Place your hands by the bottom of your rib cage.

3. Press through your hands to help lift your chin, chest, and torso.

4. Create length in the abdomen and torso to naturally bend your back.

5. Hold for as long as comfortable. Do not push through pain.

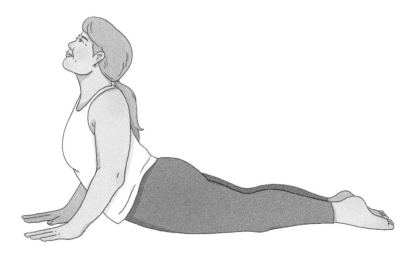

## Change It Up

- The best modification for this pose is to revert back to Sphinx pose (page 90) and place your forearms back down on the floor. If the pressure on your abdomen is too much, try placing a folded blanket under your abdomen.
- If you would like to take this further, push through your hands and try to straighten your arms as much as possible. To make it an active stretch, lift your hands off the floor completely and use your back muscles to hold yourself up.

## Remember

- Try to soften and relax the muscles in your back while you squeeze the muscles in your buttocks.
- Contraindications: back injury, pregnancy, carpal tunnel syndrome, headache, spondylitis, uncontrolled high blood pressure, and severe asthma.

# PUPPY

## Type of Stretch

- Static stretch

## Main Motion(s)

- Extension

## Affected Area(s)

- Neck, shoulders, chest

## Good For

- This stretch helps decrease tension in the neck, shoulders, chest, and spine, and it also acts as a gentle inversion. Inversions bring fresh blood to the brain that can energize you and lift your mood.

## Instructions

1. Come down onto your hands and knees in an all-fours position.

2. Walk your hands forward with your arms actively engaged.

3. Keep your hips stacked directly above your knees.

4. Allow your chest to sink down toward the floor.

5. Hold for 1 minute.

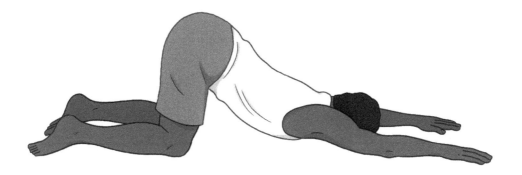

## Change It Up

- This is only hard on the knees because of the pressure put on them. Folding up a blanket under your knees can help take the pressure off and make the stretch more comfortable.
- Try resting your chin on the floor to increase the stretch in your neck and throat. Make sure it brings a feeling of length in the neck and doesn't feel uncomfortable.

## Remember

- Visualize your chest melting down toward the floor to help your back naturally bend.
- Contraindications: knee injury and frozen shoulder.

# GENTLE TWIST

## Type of Stretch

- Static stretch

## Main Motion(s)

- Twisting

## Affected Area(s)

- Back, neck

## Good For

- This stretch helps the torso and back muscles while lengthening and realigning the spine. It's a great way to relieve stress, unwind from your day, and settle into bed.

## Instructions

1. Lie down on your back with your arms out wide.

2. Bend your knees and place your feet flat on the floor.

3. Let your knees fall over to the right.

4. Turn your head to look over your left shoulder.

5. Take slow deep breaths for 1 minute before switching sides.

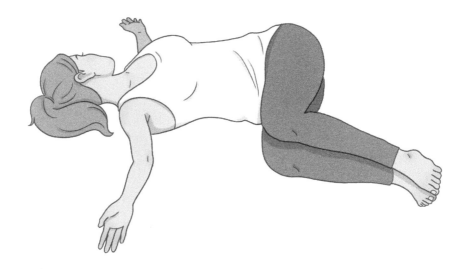

## Change It Up

- If your knees don't touch the ground, try placing a pillow between your knees and the floor to help provide more support so you can relax further.
- You can take this stretch deeper by trying to stack your hips one over the other and placing your right hand on top of your left knee with gentle pressure.

## Remember

- You can also make this a dynamic warm-up by not holding the stretch and just slowly twisting your knees from side to side. Once you get to your end range of motion, pause for a few seconds before you switch sides.
- Contraindications: recent spine, knee, or hip injury.

# SUPINE TWIST

## Type of Stretch
- Static stretch

## Main Motion(s)
- Twisting, knee and hip flexion

## Affected Area(s)
- Shoulders, spine, lower back, hips

## Good For
- Twists are known to be detoxifying and also give your abdominal organs a fresh supply of new blood. This helps lengthen and realign the spine and will improve posture and sciatica pain.

## Instructions

1. Lie down on your back.
2. Bend your right knee and pull it in toward your stomach.
3. Reach your right arm out wide.
4. Place your left hand on the outside of your right knee and pull it across your body. Place gentle pressure on the knee with your hand.
5. Place your right foot on the floor.
6. Look over your right shoulder.
7. Inhale for 4 counts, hold for 7 counts, and exhale for 8 counts.
8. Repeat on the left side.

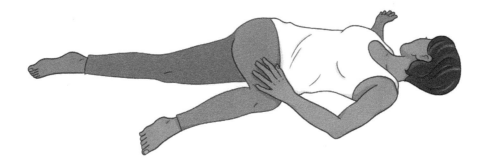

## Change It Up

- Place a pillow or folded blanket under your knee to provide more support, which will allow your body to relax deeper into the stretch.
- If you would like to intensify this stretch, keep your leg straight as you are twisting it over.

## Remember

- Make sure your shoulders stay flat on the floor, and look over your shoulder to get a full twist from your tailbone to the crown of your head.
- Contraindications: severe lumbar disc issues.

# TWISTED TWIST

## Type of Stretch

- Static stretch

## Main Motion(s)

- Twisting

## Affected Area

- Back, hips, glutes

## Good For

- This twist helps stretch the front, side, and back of the hip while elongating the spine. It can also ease menstrual and digestive cramps.

## Instructions

1. Lie down on your back with your arms out wide, knees bent, and feet on the floor.

2. Cross your right leg over your left.

3. Drop both knees over to the right as far as you can.

4. Hold for 1 minute.

5. Bring your knees back to center and then twist them to the left as far as you can.

6. Hold for 1 minute.

7. Return to center, cross your left leg over your right, and repeat.

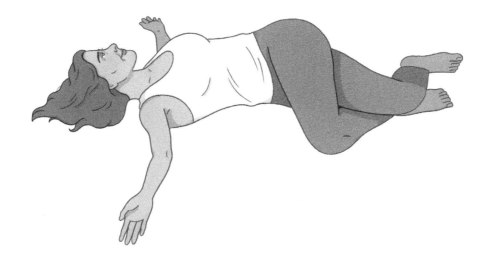

## Change It Up

- Place a pillow under your knee to give you more support and help you relax and soften deeper into the stretch.
- Try to bring your knee all the way to the floor on each side to get the deepest stretch.

## Remember

- Make sure you keep both shoulders down as you twist. If your shoulder begins to lift, you have gone too far. Just come back to center and try again.
- Contraindications: severe lumbar disc issues.

# STANDING SIDE BEND

## Type of Stretch
- Dynamic stretch
- Static stretch

## Main Motion(s)
- Side bending

## Affected Area(s)
- Obliques, shoulders

## Good For
- This stretch helps lengthen the side of your body and spine. It is an excellent stretch to do daily for your spinal health and mobility. It helps strengthen the legs and improves your posture.

## Instructions

1. Stand with your feet slightly wider than hip distance apart.
2. Reach your right arm straight overhead.
3. Place your left hand on your left outer thigh.
4. Use your left hand for support as you reach your right arm up and over.
5. Hold for 1 minute and repeat on the left side.

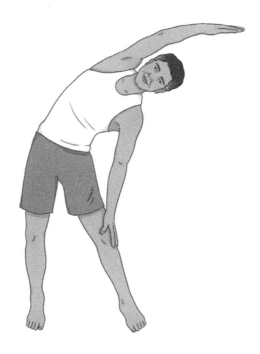

## Change It Up

- If reaching overhead is uncomfortable, try bending your arm and placing your hand behind your head as you bend to the side.
- If you don't need the support of your bottom hand, you can interlace your hands overhead before bending to the side for an active stretch. This will intensify the stretch and also engage the abdominals.

## Remember

- Focus on reaching strongly through your fingertips to help lengthen your entire side body further. For a dynamic stretch, continually switch from side to side once you have bent to your farthest point.

# BANANA

## Type of Stretch

- Static stretch

## Main Motion(s)

- Side bending

## Affected Area(s)

- Shoulders, torso, hips

## Good For

- This pose helps decompress the spine as it stretches the entire side body from your ankle all the way up to the IT band, obliques, lats, and shoulders. It's another wonderful stretch to begin or end your day with in bed.

## Instructions

1. Lie down on your back with your legs straight and arms overhead.

2. Walk your legs over to the right and cross your left ankle over the right.

3. Walk your hands over to the right.

4. Grab your left wrist and pull it over to the right more.

5. Hold for 1 minute before switching sides.

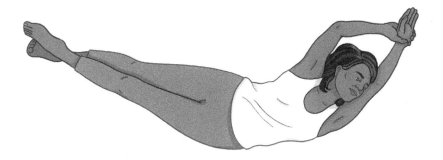

## Change It Up

- You can use a folded blanket under your heels to reduce lower back discomfort, or under the shoulders to support tight or injured shoulders that don't naturally rest on the floor.
- Think about creating more space between your hip and your rib cage to encourage more length in the side body.

## Remember

- Make sure you don't roll or twist your hips to the side. Only walk your feet over as far as you can without any other part of your body compensating.
- Contraindications: severe spinal disc or sacrum issues.

# DOORWAY PEC STRETCH

## Type of Stretch

- Static stretch

## Main Motion(s)

- Extension

## Affected Area(s)

- Chest

## Good For

- This stretch gives your body a break from computer work, and it helps improve rounded shoulders. If you are sitting a lot in your daily routine, this stretch is a great way to break up your day and correct your posture.

## Instructions

1. Stand near a doorway.

2. Reach your arm out straight and hang on to the doorway at shoulder level.

3. Take a few steps forward until you feel the stretch.

4. Then turn your toes outward from the wall and hold for 1 minute.

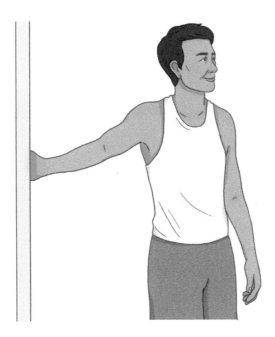

## Change It Up

- You can change this stretch by placing your hand at different levels on the doorway. Try it with your hand at hip level and with your hand as high as you can effortlessly reach.
- For another variation, do both arms at the same time by bending your elbows and placing your forearms on each side of the doorframe. Slowly step forward until you feel the stretch.

## Remember

- Many people have tight chest muscles from poor posture. If this stretch feels very intense, focus on breathing with slower exhales than inhales.

# FISH

## Type of Stretch
- Static stretch

## Main Motion(s)
- Extension

## Affected Area(s)
- Chest, back, shoulders

## Good For
- This stretch helps stimulate the thyroid and also increases lung capacity. It is the best way to reverse both rounded shoulders and forward head posture.

## Instructions

1. Sit down on the floor and place a bolster or a couple of thick pillows directly behind your spine.
2. Lie back onto the bolster.
3. Let your head hang off the end to provide a light neck stretch.
4. Reach your arms out wide.
5. Take the fullest inhalations and exhalations you can for 1 minute.

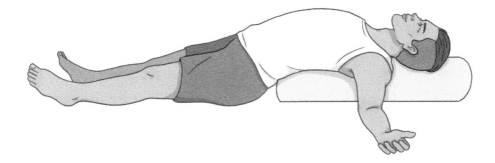

## Change It Up

- If the neck stretch is too great, you can place your head on the bolster or use a small rolled-up towel or block under the back of your head to provide a gentler stretch.
- You can also get a nice hip opening stretch by bringing the bottom of your feet together and letting your knees splay open.

## Remember

- Make sure you don't turn your head in this position. Keep your neck in line with your spine.
- Contraindications: migraine, insomnia, serious neck or lower back injury, and both uncontrolled high and low blood pressure.

# TORSO EXTENSION WITH COUNTERTOP

## Type of Stretch

- Static stretch

## Main Motion(s)

- Flexion

## Affected Area(s)

- Back, shoulders

## Good For

- This stretch helps create traction in the shoulders and back while stretching the thoracic spine. It creates a feeling of length that can help relieve tension and stress. People with lower back issues tend to love this stretch.

## Instructions

1. Stand about two feet away from the counter and place your hands on top of it.

2. Engage your core by drawing your navel to your spine to protect your back.

3. Start to lower your chest down as you reach your hips backward.

4. Think about creating length in your spine as you hold for 1 minute.

5. You can bend your knees to come out of the stretch.

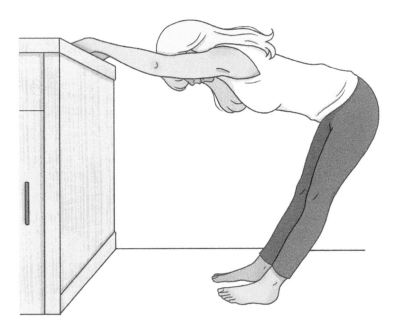

## Change It Up

- You can easily try another variation by grabbing the opposite elbows and placing them on the countertop as you extend your hips backward.
- To intensify the stretch, try doing this with your palms facing up toward the ceiling instead.

## Remember

- Imagine someone gently pulling you backward from the hips to help you lengthen your spine even further. Be careful not to lock your knees in this position.

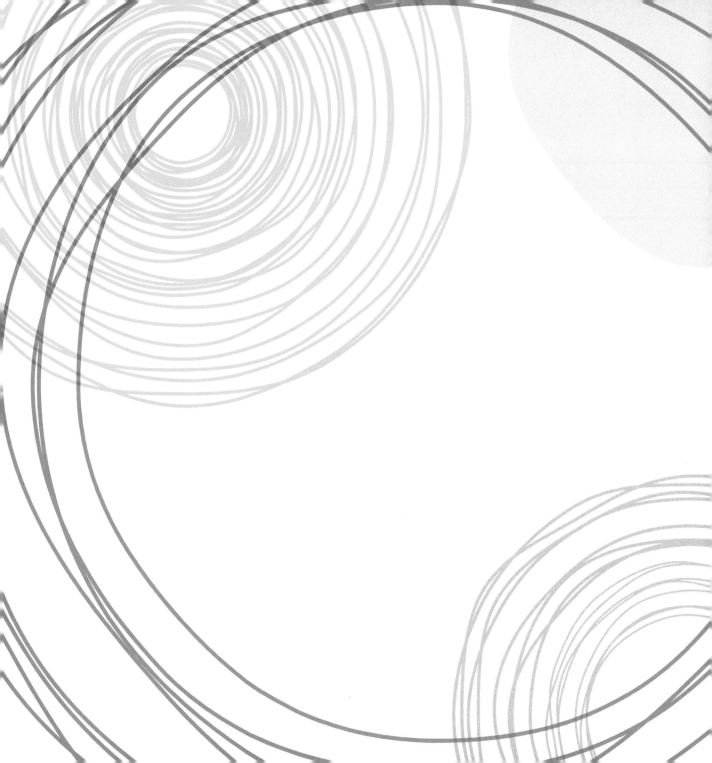

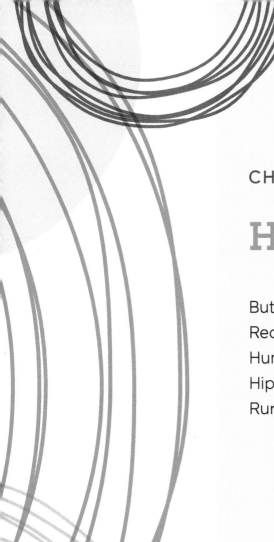

CHAPTER 8

# Hips

# BUTTERFLY

## Type of Stretch

- Dynamic stretch
- Static stretch

## Main Motion(s)

- Flexion, adduction

## Affected Area(s)

- Hips, groin, inner thighs, lower back

## Good For

- This stretch helps improve flexibility in the groin, inner thighs, hips, and lower back. It will prevent pulled muscles in the groin and will also improve hip and leg mobility.

## Instructions

1. Sit down on the floor.

2. Bring the bottom of your feet together and let your knees fall open wide.

3. Sit up tall and begin to walk your hands forward as much as you can.

4. When you reach your farthest point, you can let your spine soften and round down into the stretch.

5. Hold for 1 minute.

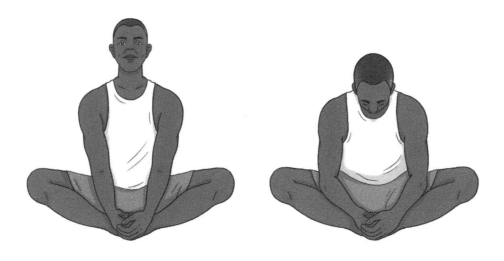

## Change It Up

- There are several variations of this stretch. Try bringing your feet closer to your groin or farther away to change the stretch. Find which distance feels like you need it the most.
- To gain a deeper hip opening and groin stretch, place your hands behind you and scoot your buttocks up toward your heels. Now, grab your ankles and use your elbows to help you push your knees down toward the mat.

## Remember

- To make this into a dynamic stretch to warm up the hips and groin, grab your ankles and let your knees gently move up and down like butterfly wings.
- Contraindications: inguinal hernia.

# RECLINING PIGEON

## Type of Stretch

- Static stretch

## Main Motion(s)

- Hip, knee, and ankle flexion; hip external rotation

## Affected Area(s)

- Piriformis, hips, glutes

## Good For

- This stretch is very therapeutic and can help relieve an impinged piriformis and sciatica pain. It opens up the hips and relieves deep tension stored in the glutes and lower back.

## Instructions

1. Lie down on your back with your knees bent and feet on the floor.

2. Cross your right ankle over your left thigh.

3. Lift your left foot up off the floor as you reach your hands around your left thigh.

4. Pull your thigh in toward you as far as you can and flex both ankles.

5. Hold for at least 1 minute before switching sides.

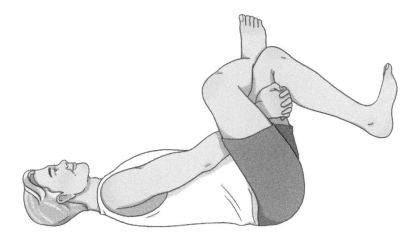

## Change It Up

- If you can't easily reach your thigh, use a strap around the back of your thigh to help you pull your leg closer. If you can easily reach your thigh, try grabbing your shin to deepen the stretch.
- You can both release and deepen the stretch by gently rocking the leg slightly from side to side. Keep your back down so you don't roll all the way over to your side.

## Remember

- Try to keep your crossed knee opening wide to help increase the inner thigh stretch.

# HURDLER'S STRETCH

## Type of Stretch

- Static stretch

## Main Motion(s)

- Flexion

## Affected Area(s)

- Hamstrings, groin, hips, lower back

## Good For

- As the name implies, this is a great stretch for athletes who run hurdles! It can also help increase hamstring flexibility while opening the hip and groin.

## Instructions

1. Sit down on the floor with your legs straight out in front of you.

2. Bend your right knee and bring your right foot to your left inner thigh.

3. Sit up tall and walk your hands down your left leg.

4. Once you are at your farthest point, soften and relax into the stretch.

5. Hold for 1 minute before switching sides.

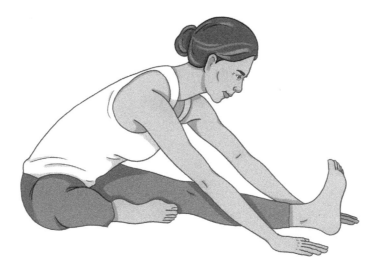

## Change It Up

- Place a pillow under your bent knee to keep it supported. You can also use a strap around the bottom of your foot to help you pull yourself deeper into the stretch.
- You can fold over your bent leg instead of the straight leg to get a different stretch in the same position.

## Remember

- Close your eyes and connect with your hamstring muscle. Imagine the tension leaving your hamstring every time you exhale.
- Contraindications: pregnancy, severe disc issues; those with knee issues should place support under both knees.

# HIP CIRCLES

### Type of Stretch

- Dynamic stretch

### Main Motion(s)

- Rotation

### Affected Area(s)

- Lower back, hips, hamstrings

### Good For

- This is a great total body warm-up before any type of activity. The circular movement helps lubricate the joints in the hips and lower back, making it wonderful for those with arthritis and joint replacements.

### Instructions

1. Stand with your feet slightly wider than hip width apart with your hands on your hips.

2. Begin to move your hips in a clockwise circle.

3. Use your head and torso to counterbalance your hips movements and let them move in the opposite direction of your hips.

4. Do 10 to 20 circles and then switch directions.

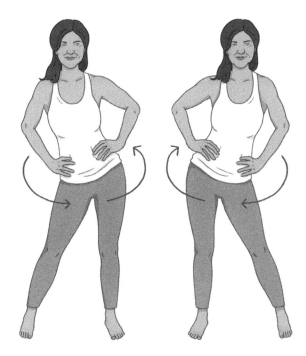

## Change It Up

- Try starting off with very small circles and let them slowly become larger and larger. Notice what size circles feel the best in your body.
- Use your hands on your hips to help you push the hips around in bigger circles.

## Remember

- Notice which part of the circle feels like it has more tension or less mobility. Focus on moving back and forth through that particular range of motion and then return to the full circles again.

# RUNNER'S LUNGE

## Type of Stretch

- Active stretch
- Static stretch

## Main Motion(s)

- Flexion, extension

## Affected Area(s)

- Hips, psoas, lower back

## Good For

- This stretch helps reverse our seated posture and alleviates lower back pain that stems from tight psoas muscles. It is excellent for runners, cyclists, and athletes.

## Instructions

1. Come down to a kneeling position.
2. Step your right foot forward into a low lunge.
3. Make sure your front knee and ankle are in a straight line.
4. Allow your hips to sink forward.
5. You can rest your hands on top of your leg or reach down to the floor.
6. Hold for at least 1 minute before switching sides.

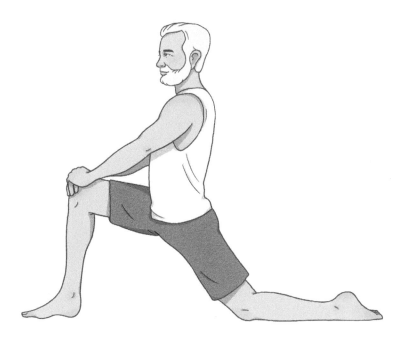

## Change It Up

- Place your back knee on a blanket if it feels like too much pressure. You can also place blocks on each side of your front leg so you can rest your hands and relax your shoulders even if you can't reach the floor.
- You can turn this into an active stretch by lifting your back knee off the floor and pushing back through your heel to flex the foot.

## Remember

- Reaching your arms up by your ears will create a much deeper stretch from your bottom knee all the way up your torso to your arms.

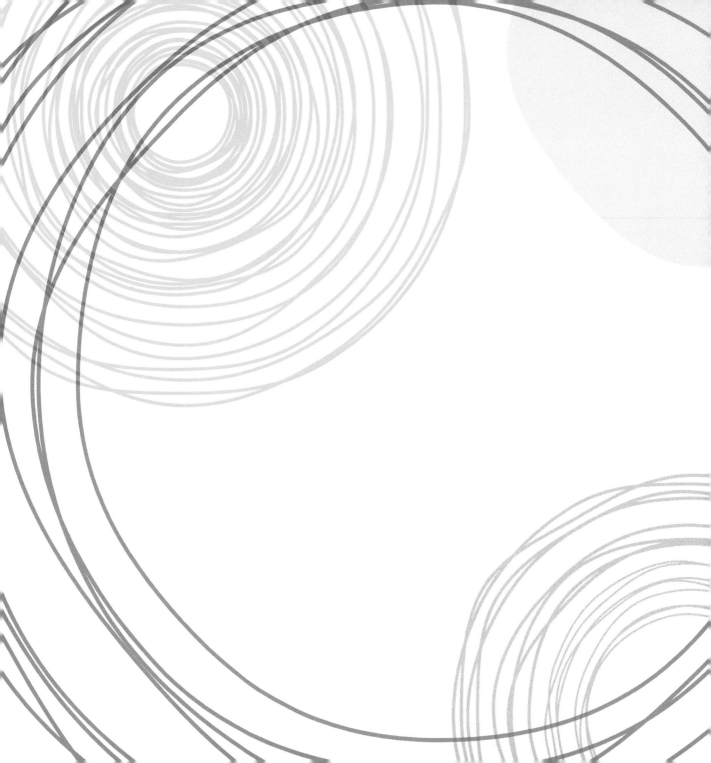

CHAPTER 9

# Upper Legs and Knees

# STANDING QUAD STRETCH

## Type of Stretch

- Static stretch

## Main Motion(s)

- Knee flexion

## Affected Area(s)

- Quadriceps

## Good For

- Most of our daily activities are quadriceps dominant, from walking up stairs to the sports and activities we engage in. This exercise can help stretch out your quadriceps and provide relief from knee pain. It's also ideal after a lower body workout.

## Instructions

1. Stand with your feet about hip width apart.

2. Bend your right knee and reach your left hand back to grab your right ankle.

3. Pull your heel as close as you can to your buttocks.

4. Bring your knees together and push your hips forward.

5. Hold for 1 minute before switching sides.

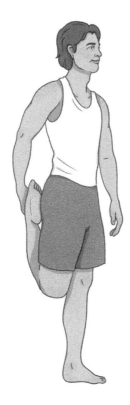

## Change It Up

- If you struggle to reach your foot, try placing your knee on a chair and using a strap around your ankle to help you pull the heel toward your buttocks.
- To make this stretch more challenging, reach back to grab the ankle with your same hand.

## Remember

- Keep a small bend in the knee of your standing leg so you don't lock it. Try to tuck your tailbone under and push your hips forward to get the most out of it.

# STANDING FORWARD FOLD

### Type of Stretch

- Static stretch

### Main Motion(s)

- Flexion

### Affected Area(s)

- Hamstrings, lower back

### Good For

- This is an intense hamstring stretch that will help calm your mind and reduce stress, anxiety, and fatigue. It offers a wonderful inversion to help oxygenate the brain.

### Instructions

1. Stand with your feet together.
2. Bend over and reach down for your toes.
3. Try to lengthen your spine as you reach down for the floor.
4. Hold for at least 1 minute, focusing on slow exhales.

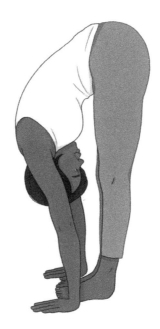

## Change It Up

- Bend your knees in order to modify the stretch for tight hamstrings. If you can't reach the floor, rest your hands on a yoga block or chair placed in front of you.
- If you would like to make the stretch more challenging, grab opposite elbows to help gravity assist you. Another variation you can try is to cross one ankle in front of the other before you reach down.

## Remember

- Imagine wearing a lead bicycle helmet that is weighing you down, creating traction in your spine. This visualization will help you create more space between the vertebrae and will allow you to reach farther.
- Contraindications: uncontrolled high blood pressure, glaucoma, acid reflux, and disc issues.

# SEATED FORWARD FOLD

## Type of Stretch

- Static stretch

## Main Motion(s)

- Flexion

## Affected Area(s)

- Hamstrings, lower back

## Good For

- This pose will help stretch the hamstrings and lower back while being highly therapeutic for high blood pressure, infertility, and insomnia. As with most forward bends, it can also help soothe a headache or anxiety.

## Instructions

1. Sit down on the floor with your legs straight out in front of you.

2. Sit up tall and walk your hands forward on the floor.

3. When you can no longer walk your hands any farther, exhale and soften into the stretch.

4. Hold for at least 1 minute.

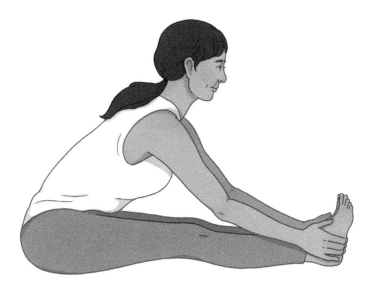

## Change It Up

- There are many ways to modify this stretch. Try sitting on a folded blanket to elevate your hips, placing a rolled-up blanket under your knees, or using a strap around the bottom of your feet to help pull yourself forward.
- If you would like to make this more challenging, try placing a block at the bottom of your feet and reaching your hands around it.

## Remember

- Always try to think about creating length in your spine as you reach forward rather than rounding down immediately.
- Contraindications: severe back injury, diarrhea, and asthma.

# SIDE LUNGE

## Type of Stretch

- Active stretch
- Dynamic stretch
- Static stretch

## Main Motion(s)

- Flexion, abduction

## Affected Area(s)

- Hips, groin, hamstrings, glutes

## Good For

- This stretch is ideal to warm up for or recover from side-to-side movements. It helps stretch and strengthen the adductors while also strengthening the glutes. It can also relieve back pain and sciatica issues.

## Instructions

1. Stand with your feet wide apart and toes turned slightly outward.
2. Bend your right knee at a 90-degree angle while keeping the left leg out straight and wide.
3. Bring your hands down to the floor to support yourself.
4. Hold for 1 minute before switching sides.

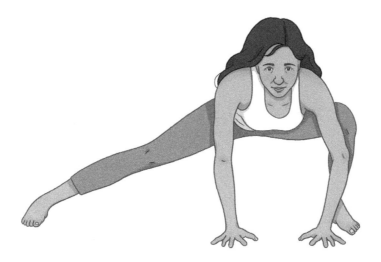

## Change It Up

- Use blocks in front of you if your hands can't reach the floor. It can also be helpful to lift the toes of your straight leg off the floor.
- Turn this into a dynamic stretch by continually moving from side to side as soon as you find your end range of motion. Make this an active stretch by lifting your hands up into the air as you hold the stretch.

## Remember

- Try to keep your spine straight and don't round over in this stretch.
- Contraindications: current hip, knee, or ankle injuries.

# SEATED STRADDLE

## Type of Stretch
- PNF stretch
- Static stretch

## Main Motion(s)
- Abduction, flexion

## Affected Area(s)
- Inner thighs, hamstrings

## Good For
- This pose helps stretch the hamstrings and inner thighs. It can also be therapeutic for sacroiliac (SI) joint issues.

## Instructions

1. Sit down on the floor with your legs spread out wide.

2. Place your hands on the floor in front of you.

3. Walk your hands forward with a straight spine.

4. When you reach your farthest point, exhale and soften down into the stretch.

5. Hold for at least 1 minute.

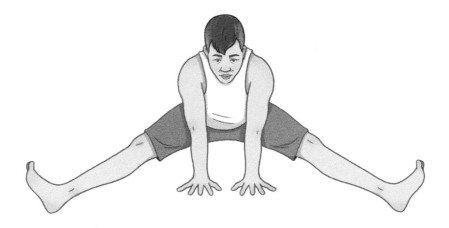

## Change It Up

- You can sit on a thick folded blanket to elevate your hips so your posture will become easier. Placing a stack of pillows or a bolster in front of you to rest on can also help you relax.
- Turn this into a PNF stretch by contracting the quadriceps for 6 seconds and then reaching farther. If you can place your torso flat on the floor, you can bend your knees slightly and slide your arms under them to take the stretch further.

## Remember

- Make sure you keep both your knees and toes pointed directly up toward the sky.
- Contraindications: Keep your knees slightly bent if you have knee, back, hip, or groin issues.

# STANDING STRADDLE

## Type of Stretch

- Static stretch

## Main Motion(s)

- Flexion

## Affected Area(s)

- Hamstrings, inner thighs

## Good For

- This pose helps stretch the inner thighs, elongates the spine, and gives you an inversion too! Every part of the nervous system is stimulated by this position.

## Instructions

1. Stand up tall with your feet spread wide apart.

2. Place your hands on your hips and fold forward as far as you can with a flat back.

3. Reach down to the floor as you lengthen your spine.

4. Hold for at least 1 minute.

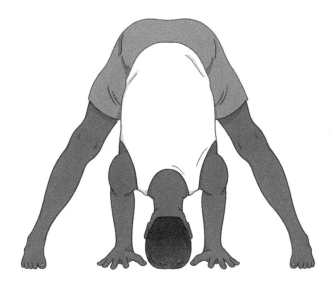

## Change It Up

- If you can't reach the floor, place your hands on blocks instead.
- If your head is close to the floor, you can walk your hands through the space between your legs to pull yourself deeper into the stretch.

## Remember

- Keep your ankles stable, and be careful that your feet don't roll outward. Just notice the difference between putting your weight in your heels versus your toes, and then try to press evenly through both feet.
- Contraindications: Those with uncontrolled high blood pressure, back issues, and reflux issues should not extend their torso below hip level. Place your hands on your thighs or a chair in front of you for support.

# IT BAND FOLD

## Type of Stretch

- Static stretch

## Main Motion(s)

- Flexion, rotation

## Affected Area(s)

- IT band, hamstrings

## Good For

- The IT band is a ligament, not a muscle, so we can't actually stretch it, but this exercise will help stretch the connecting muscles. This is a great stretch to do after a run or another athletic activity, and it can help ease IT band syndrome, knee pain, and hip pain.

## Instructions

1. Stand up tall with your feet hip width apart.

2. Bend your right knee slightly.

3. Hinge forward from the hips and reach both hands to the floor.

4. Reach your left arm up into the air and allow your torso to twist.

5. Hold for 1 minute before switching sides.

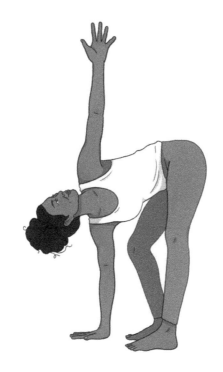

## Change It Up

- If you can't reach the floor or your fingertips are only grazing it, place a block on the floor to rest your hand on instead.
- To deepen the twist, place your hand on the ankle of your straight leg.

## Remember

- Close your eyes and connect with what you are feeling in your body. Focus on letting any tension or discomfort leave your muscles every time you exhale.
- Contraindications: Those with wrist, knee, or hip issues should use a block or chair under their bottom hand for support. Those with neck issues should keep their head neutral or facing down.

# HALF SPLIT

## Type of Stretch
- PNF stretch
- Static stretch

## Main Motion(s)
- Flexion

## Affected Area(s)
- Hamstrings

## Good For
- This is a more intense hamstring stretch that is great for working on front splits and recovering from lower body workouts.

## Instructions

1. Come down into a kneeling position.
2. Extend your right leg straight in front of you.
3. Fold forward over your right leg, bringing your hands to the floor.
4. Focus on slow exhales as you hold the stretch for 1 minute.
5. Switch sides.

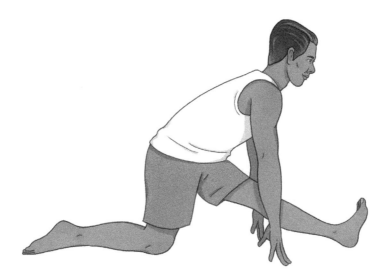

## Change It Up

- If you feel like you can barely reach your fingertips to the floor, place blocks under your hands so you don't have to fold quite so far. You can also place a blanket under your back knee for extra cushioning.
- Flex your foot up toward your shin to intensify the stretch. For the PNF variation, simply contract the quadriceps of your straight leg for 6 seconds and then relax them to move deeper into the stretch.

## Remember

- Our body tries to compensate to make things easier for us. Make sure your back knee stays in a straight line below your hip and your front leg stays straight.

# SINGLE LEG HAMSTRING STRETCH

**Type of Stretch**
- PNF stretch
- Static stretch

**Main Motion(s)**
- Hip flexion

**Affected Area(s)**
- Hamstrings

**Good For**
- This is the best stretch for increasing flexibility in your hamstrings. It can also help relieve lower back pain that stems from tight hamstrings.

**Instructions**

1. Lie down on your back and place a strap around your right foot.
2. Lift your leg straight into the air as high as you can.
3. Slide your hands down the strap to rest your elbows on the floor.
4. Hold for 1 to 5 minutes before switching sides.

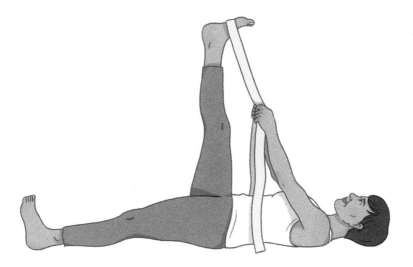

## Change It Up

- If you have extremely tight hamstrings, bend the knee of your resting leg and place your foot on the floor.
- For a PNF stretch, you can push down and resist into the strap for 6 seconds before you exhale to pull the leg back into a deeper stretch. Repeat 3 times.

## Remember

- Try rocking your leg slightly from side to side to find the angle you are tightest in. Spend some time holding your leg at this angle in addition to straight up and down.

# SINGLE LEG SUPINE STRADDLE

## Type of Stretch

- PNF stretch
- Static stretch

## Main Motion(s)

- Abduction

## Affected Area(s)

- Inner thighs, groin

## Good For

- This stretch helps increase mobility in the hips and stretches the inner thighs and groin. These muscles are tight on most people because our daily activities do not include this movement.

## Instructions

1. Lie on your back and place a strap around the bottom of your right foot.

2. Reach your left arm straight out on the floor and lift your right leg straight up into the air.

3. Try to keep your left hip down as you bring your right leg out as wide as you can.

4. Hold for at least 1 minute.

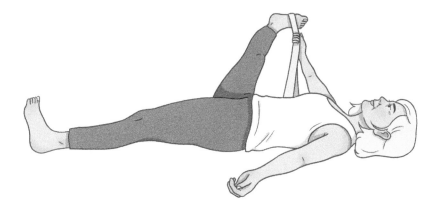

## Change It Up

- Lowering the angle of your leg below hip level will make this stretch easier; lifting it above hip level will make it more intense.
- For a PNF stretch, push your leg downward into the strap for 6 seconds, then quickly stop resisting and lift the leg back up as high as you can while you exhale. Repeat 3 times.

## Remember

- Try keeping your free hand on your hip. This tactile sensation will help you keep the hip grounded.

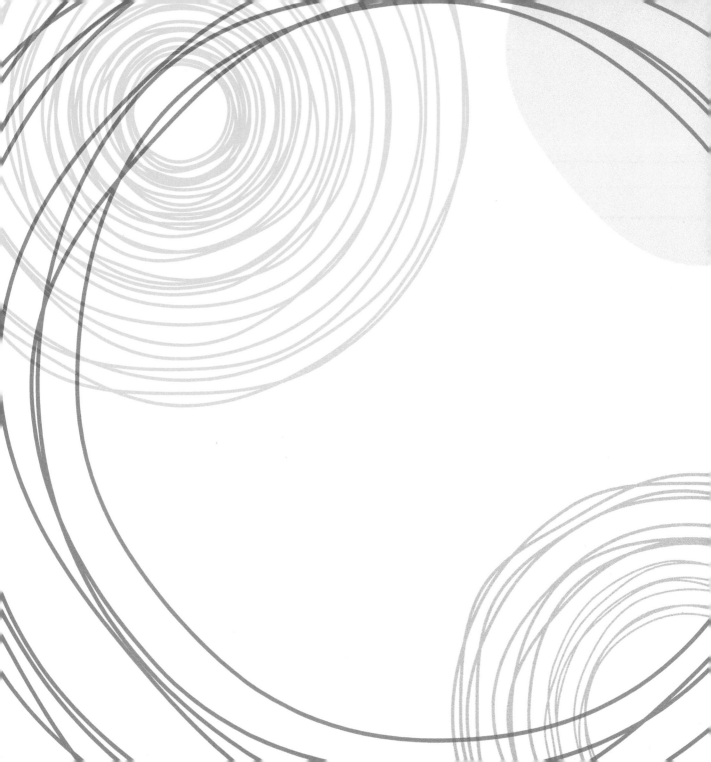

# Lower Legs, Feet, and Ankles

# POINT AND FLEX

## Type of Stretch

- Dynamic stretch

## Main Motion(s)

- Dorsiflexion, plantar flexion

## Affected Area(s)

- Feet, calves, shins

## Good For

- This is a gentle stretch that can be great for rehabilitating the ankle after injuries, but it will also help prevent them from happening too.

## Instructions

1. You can sit in a chair or on the floor.
2. Stretch your right leg out in front of you.
3. Point your toes down to the floor and hold for 5 seconds.
4. Flex your toes up toward your shin and hold for 5 seconds.
5. Repeat for 5 to 10 rounds before switching sides.

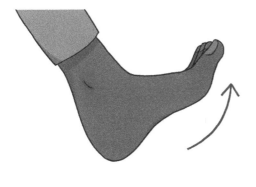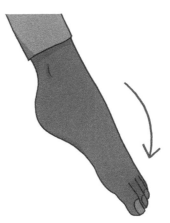

## Change It Up

- You can wrap a towel or resistance band around the ball of your foot to push against as a way to help you feel more supported and pull deeper into the stretch.
- You could do this stretch standing up too, but have something nearby to help you balance. Rock back onto your heels, lift your toes up, and then rock onto your toes and lift your heels up.

## Remember

- You are trying to find your full range of motion in the ankle. Try to point and flex to the end range and hold it there for the full 5 seconds.

# TOWEL PULLS

## Type of Stretch

- Static stretch

## Main Motion(s)

- Dorsiflexion

## Affected Area(s)

- Calves

## Good For

- This is a common physical therapy exercise for ankle injuries because it not only stretches the calf, but it also helps strengthen the ankle.

## Instructions

1. Sit on the floor with your legs straight out in front of you.

2. Bend your left leg in.

3. Wrap a strap or towel around the ball of your right foot.

4. Pull your toes toward your head while keeping your heel down.

5. Hold for 1 minute and repeat on the other side.

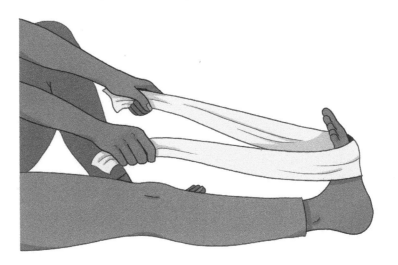

## Change It Up

- If you find it uncomfortable to sit on the floor, try placing a pillow or bolster under your buttocks. This elevates the hips and modifies the stretch on the hamstrings to help you reach forward with more ease.
- You can turn this into a PNF stretch by resisting against the towel for 6 seconds and then relaxing deeper into the stretch. Repeat 3 times and hold the final stretch for 1 minute.

## Remember

- Try to keep the muscles in your hands, arms, and shoulders as relaxed as possible so you don't create more tension in your body.

# LEG SWINGS

## Type of Stretch

- Dynamic stretch

## Main Motion(s)

- Hip flexion and extension

## Affected Area(s)

- Hips, hamstrings

## Good For

- This stretch helps prepare the lower body for movement. It quickly improves circulation and mobility in the hip joint. It can also be a great break between lower body exercises to help push the lactic acid out.

## Instructions

1. Stand with your feet hip width apart. You may want to be near a chair or wall to help you balance.

2. Reach your right leg forward.

3. Swing it back and forth like a pendulum.

4. Repeat 10 to 20 times per side.

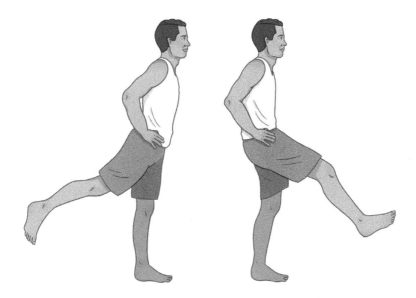

## Change It Up

- Changing the pace helps change the intensity and benefits of the stretch. Play with your cadence by slowing your swings down and speeding them up to find what feels best.
- You can do this stretch standing on a yoga block to give your leg more clearance. Place the block near the wall so you can use it for support, and really let your leg hang down as long as possible while swinging.

## Remember

- Keep your spine upright and don't let the rest of your body overcompensate for the swinging movement. You want your leg to reach the point that's farthest in front of you and behind you without your torso shifting positions.

# TOE SPREAD

## Type of Stretch
- Dynamic stretch

## Main Motion(s)
- Abduction

## Affected Area(s)
- Feet, toes

## Good For
- This stretch helps increase the mobility of the foot and can also help improve your balance. Our toes spend most of their lives crammed into a shoe. This stretch lets them find their proper alignment again.

## Instructions

1. Sit in any position that is comfortable for you.

2. Spread your toes as wide apart as you can and hold for 5 seconds.

3. Relax your toes and repeat 10 times.

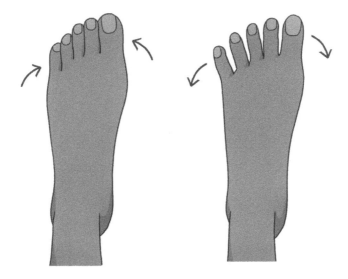

## Change It Up

- If you are struggling to create space between your toes, you can try doing this manually by reaching down and using your fingers to help pull your toes apart.
- Challenge yourself to see how many seconds you can hold your toes apart for. This will help improve the stretch but can also help strengthen the muscles in the foot.

## Remember

- The more difficult this is for you, the more your body really needs this stretch. Don't overlook the importance of foot health. The way we walk affects every joint in our body, from the ankles up to the neck.

# ANKLE ALPHABET

### Type of Stretch

- Dynamic stretch

### Main Motion(s)

- Rotation

### Affected Area(s)

- Feet, ankles, calves

### Good For

- This stretch moves the ankle joint in every possible range of motion. This makes it a wonderful exercise for rehabilitating the ankle or simply warming it up before an activity.

### Instructions

1. Sit on the floor with your leg straight out in front of you.

2. Place a rolled-up towel or pillow under your knee.

3. Begin to write the alphabet with your foot.

4. Switch feet once you have gone from A to Z.

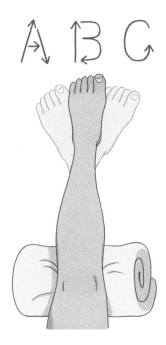

## Change It Up

- If sitting on the floor is uncomfortable, you can do this stretch while sitting in a chair instead. If the 26 letters of the alphabet feel like too much, you could try writing your name instead.
- You can loop a long resistance band around the ball of your foot to provide extra resistance as you are pushing away from the body and better leverage when you are pulling the foot toward your body.

## Remember

- Don't lose sight of your posture while you are focused on your ankle. Sit up tall and make sure your body is in a comfortable and relaxed position.

# ANKLE CIRCLES

## Type of Stretch

- Dynamic stretch

## Main Motion(s)

- Rotation

## Affected Area(s)

- Feet, ankles, calves

## Good For

- This stretch helps lubricate the ankle joint so it can move with more freedom. This is a great warm-up for any standing activity and can help relieve arthritis. It is also an excellent choice for ankle rehabilitation.

## Instructions

1. Sitting in a chair, extend your right leg out in front of you.

2. Begin making large circles with your foot in a clockwise direction.

3. After making 10 to 15 circles, switch directions.

4. Do 10 to 15 circles counterclockwise and then switch legs.

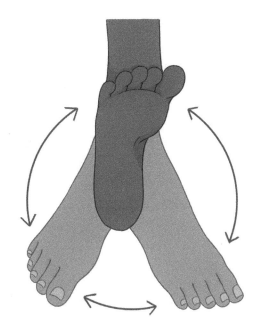

### Change It Up

- Notice if there is any part of your circle that doesn't move quite so well. Try working on just that part of the circle, back and forth 10 times, and then try the full circle again.
- Think about the circle like the face of a clock. Try to hold your ankle in the stretch for 5 seconds at every number on the clock face from 1 to 12 in both a clockwise and counterclockwise direction.

### Remember

- Moving quickly is great for getting the ankle joint warmed up, but you have to move slowly to truly find your largest range of motion.

# WALL CALF STRETCH

## Type of Stretch

- Static stretch

## Main Motion(s)

- Dorsiflexion

## Affected Area(s)

- Calves

## Good For

- This is a more intense calf stretch that is easy to do anywhere after being active! It's highly important to stretch your calves because they are in a slightly contracted position just from the shoes we wear.

## Instructions

1. Stand a few inches away from a wall or the bottom of a staircase.

2. Place your right toes up against the wall or bottom step with your heel on the floor.

3. Flex your foot as much as you can as you lean forward slightly.

4. Hold for 1 minute before switching sides.

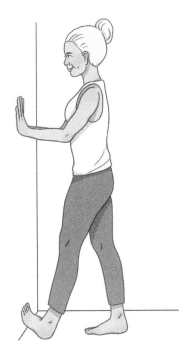

## Change It Up

- The higher up you place your toes, the more intense the stretch becomes. If you need to decrease the intensity, just place your toes slightly lower and try again.
- You can also do this stretch while standing on a curb or step by just letting your heel hang off. Make sure you have something to hold on to if you get off balance.

## Remember

- You can add variety to any calf stretch by changing the angle of your foot. Try doing this stretch with your foot straight, turned out, and turned in slightly.

# RUNNER'S CALF STRETCH

## Type of Stretch

- Static stretch

## Main Motion(s)

- Dorsiflexion

## Affected Area(s)

- Calves

## Good For

- This exercise helps stretch out the calf muscles and is often done directly after engaging in athletic activity since you can do it standing up and on your way out. As the name implies, this is a popular stretch for runners!

## Instructions

1. Stand slightly less than an arm's distance away from a wall.

2. Step your left leg forward and right leg back, keeping your feet parallel.

3. Bend your left knee and push down through your right heel.

4. Hold for at least 1 minute before switching sides.

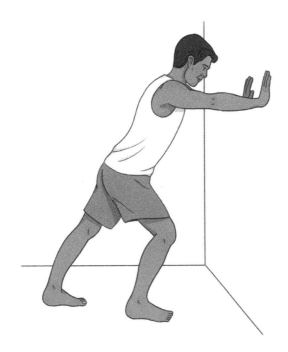

## Change It Up

- If you want to make this stretch gentler, just shorten your stance and don't step back quite as far. Experiment and find what distance between your feet provides you with the best stretch.
- Keep your core engaged with your arms straight and press through the wall to help isometrically strengthen your core, arms, and shoulders while you stretch.

## Remember

- Try to keep your body in alignment by visualizing it in a perfect diagonal line. The calf muscle is considered a postural muscle because it has to be engaged for long periods without fatiguing. This makes it an important muscle to stretch daily.

# ALL-FOURS CALF STRETCH

## Type of Stretch
- Static stretch

## Main Motion(s)
- Dorsiflexion

## Affected Area(s)
- Calves

## Good For
- This pose helps stretch the calf muscle and is ideal to do after standing activities. Tight calves can contribute to a variety of foot issues, such as plantar fasciitis. Stretching your calves can help relieve this foot pain.

## Instructions

1. Come down onto your hands and knees in an all-fours position.

2. Extend your right leg straight back, placing your foot on the floor.

3. Exhale as you push back through your heel to deeply flex the ankle.

4. Hold for 1 minute before switching sides.

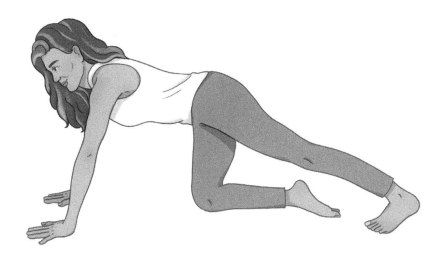

## Change It Up

- There are a variety of modifications to try if you have wrist issues. You can do this stretch while holding on to dumbbells or while resting down on your forearms. You can also place your hands on yoga blocks to take some of the pressure off.
- Use this time to strengthen your core by drawing your belly button up toward your spine. Turn this into a dynamic stretch by performing it quickly 10 to 15 times.

## Remember

- Make sure you don't create tension in your neck and shoulders. Push firmly through your hands so you don't sink into your shoulder joints.

# INVERTED V

## Type of Stretch

- Static stretch

## Main Motion(s)

- Shoulder and hip flexion

## Affected Area

- Shoulders, back, hamstrings, calves

## Good For

- This is a great total body stretch, and it can also help isometrically strengthen the upper body. The inversion will make blood rush to your head, which gives you a boost of fresh oxygen that will help shift your mood.

## Instructions

1. Start off in a push-up position.

2. Shift your hips and buttocks into the air to make an inverted V with your body.

3. Broaden your shoulder blades wide across your back.

4. Push down through your heels.

5. Keep your head and neck aligned with your spine.

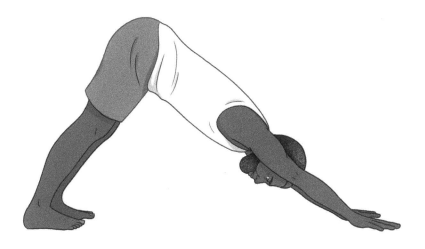

## Change It Up

- This can be an intense calf stretch. Alternate bending your knees and focusing on pushing the heel of your straight leg to the ground. You can pedal back and forth or hold it.
- If you want an extra challenge, try lifting one leg straight into the air as high as you can! Make sure you try both sides.

## Remember

- Spread your fingers wide apart and push down into your thumbs and index fingers to help take pressure off your wrists.
- Contraindications: high blood pressure, carpal tunnel syndrome, and late-term pregnancy.

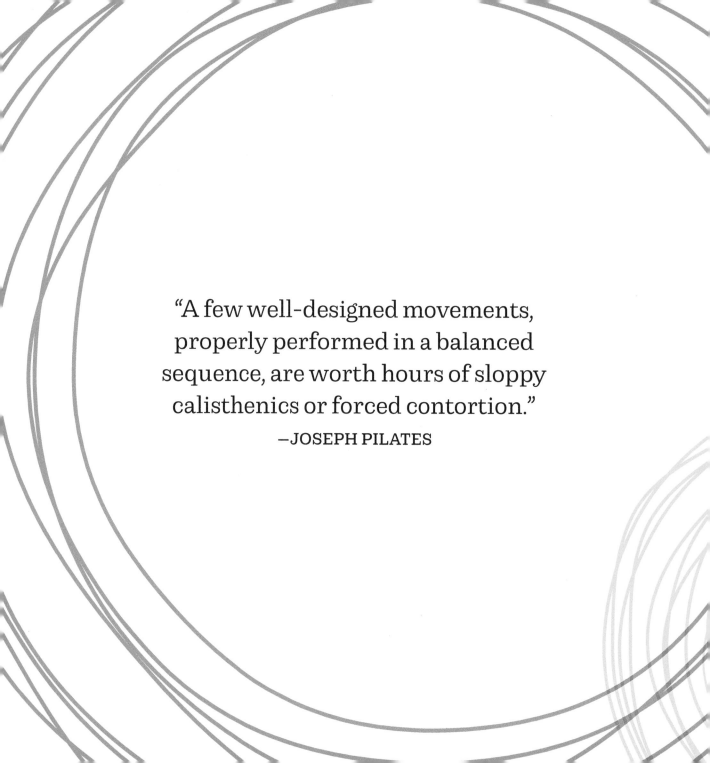

"A few well-designed movements, properly performed in a balanced sequence, are worth hours of sloppy calisthenics or forced contortion."

—JOSEPH PILATES

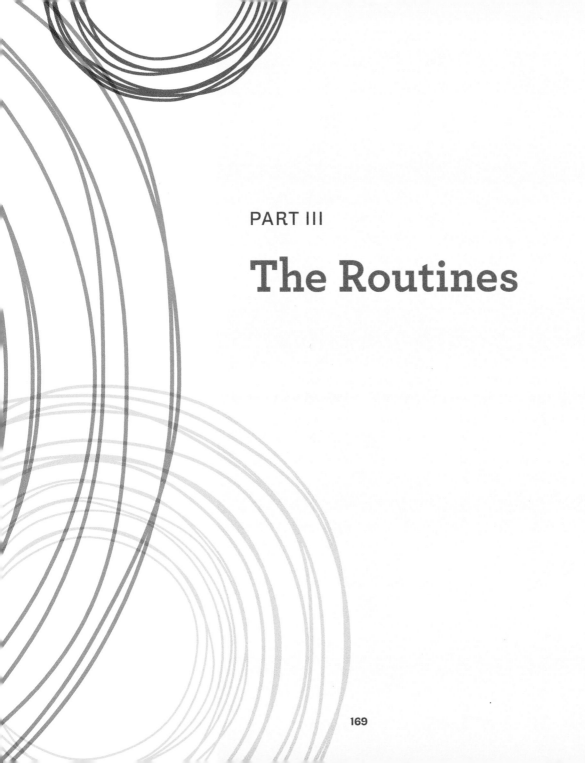

PART III

# The Routines

# HOW TO USE THE ROUTINES

Short stretching routines can be used for a wide variety of purposes. Combining different stretches into a specific routine gives the individual stretches a more profound compound benefit. I created the following stretch routines with a specific order in mind so that the first stretch is helping the body prepare for the next one and so on. This is one reason routines and sequences can be transformational when planned properly. If you did these routines in reverse, they would feel much different because your body wouldn't be warmed up properly for each successive stretch. For this reason, I don't recommend doing these sequences in a different order than listed.

The following 35 sequences will help you find the essential stretching routines you need to address your unique flexibility and mobility needs both safely and efficiently. The sequences are clearly laid out with illustrations for each stretch, instructions for how long to hold the stretches, and guidance on the best breathing technique for each routine, along with a helpful tip to remember. There are sequences for everything from going for a walk to lifting your mood.

All the routines can be completed in 10 minutes or less, which is all the time you need to get the maximum benefits out of stretching. It is so easy to fit these routines into your everyday activities, and I know they will improve the quality of your life in new and surprising ways. Remember that the more often you stretch, the more benefits you will gain. Start thinking about how many stretching routines you can fit into your day. In chapter 16 you will learn how to create your own routines so you can address your specific needs even better.

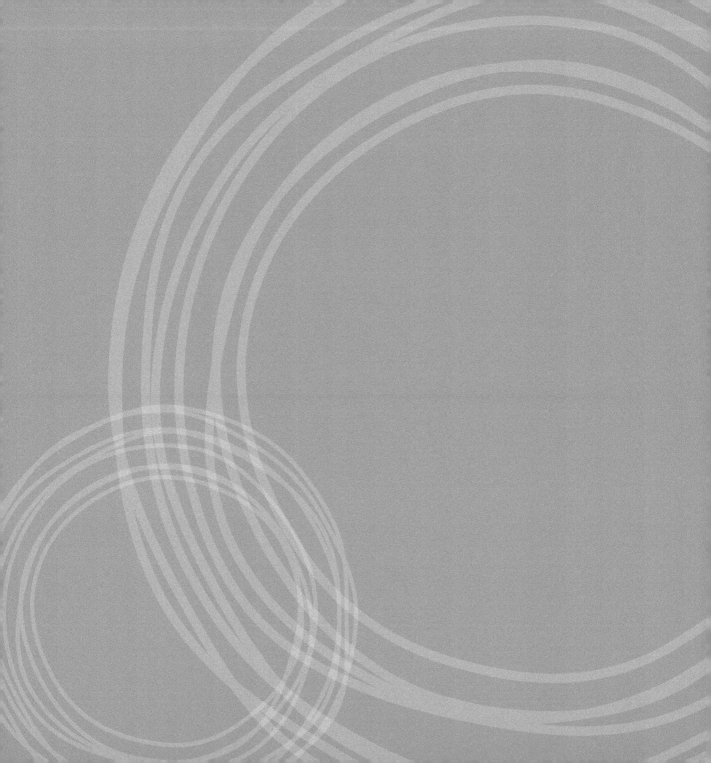

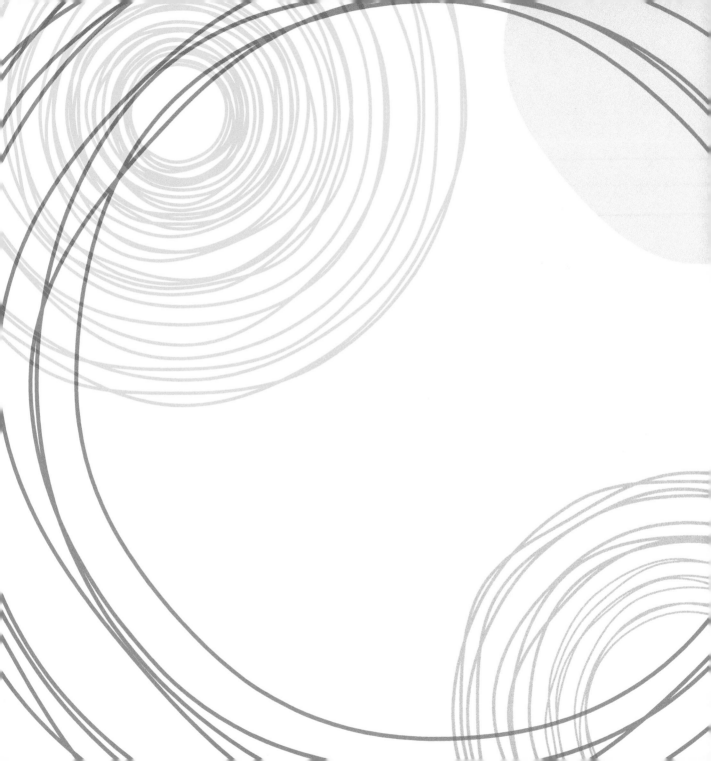

CHAPTER 11

# Everyday Activities

# WALKING

## Good For

- This is a great warm-up routine for any standing activity. It will help you get the blood flowing and the muscles warmed up for both standing and walking.

## Routine

1. Shoulder Shrug and Release (page 48)
2. Arm Swings (page 60)
3. Leg Swings (page 152)
4. Standing Side Bend (page 102)

## Holding and Repetitions

- Perform the dynamic stretch variation for each exercise. Continue to move in and out of each stretch for 1 full minute.

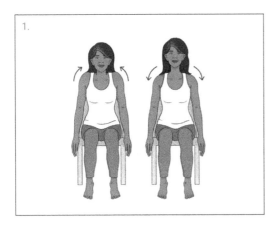

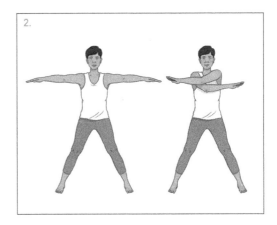

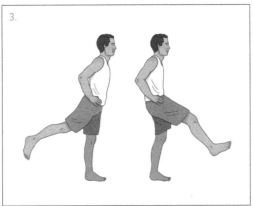

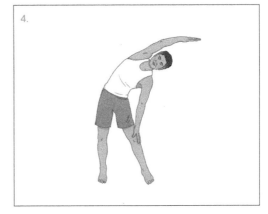

## Remember

- Try to connect your movement and breathing together so you are inhaling as you transition into the stretch and exhaling in your end range of motion.

# OFFICE BREAK

## Good For

- We place a lot of wear and tear on our bodies just by sitting in uncomfortable positions all day. If you are sitting a lot, the more stretch breaks you can take, the better!

## Routine

1. Doorway Pec Stretch (page 106)
2. Back Scratch (page 58)
3. Runner's Lunge (page 122)
4. Neck Retractions (page 44)
5. Shoulder Shrug and Release (page 48)

## Holding and Repetitions

- Try box breathing, using the 5-count example that appears on page x. Repeat this breathing cycle three times during each stretch to hold for 1 minute.

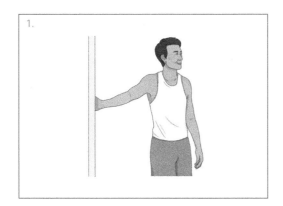

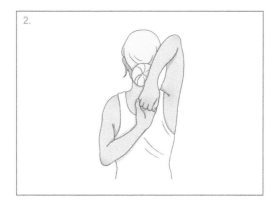

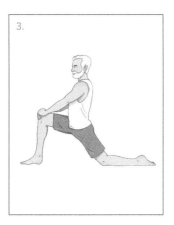

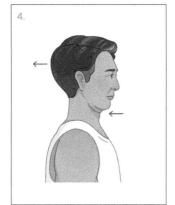

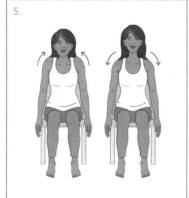

## Remember

- You don't even need to leave your office for this one, but you have to stand up from your chair to get started and sit back down to finish it off.

# GARDENING

## Good For

- Gardening can be great for the heart and mind, but it can be hard on the body! This sequence will help you prepare to squat, bend, and reach.

## Routine

1. Quadruped Cat Cow (page 84) or Seated Cat Cow (page 82)

2. Runner's Lunge (page 122)

3. Half Split (page 140)

4. Seated Twist (page 88)

## Holding and Repetitions

- Take your time and breathe slowly during each stretch for 60 to 90 seconds.

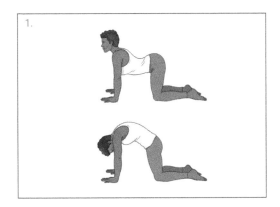

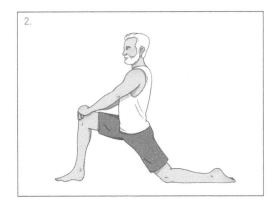

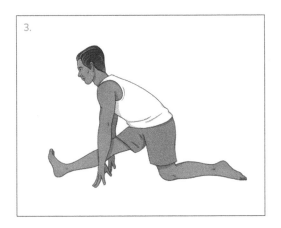

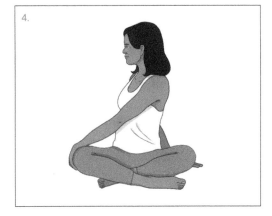

## Remember

- The reason dynamic stretching isn't necessary here, even though this is a warm-up before an activity, is because gardening doesn't require power from the muscles. You could use this routine after gardening too!

# MORNING STRETCH

## Good For

- Our spine compresses each night while we sleep and can take about 45 minutes to come back to its normal length. This sequence bends the spine in all six ranges to help prepare the body for the day.

## Routine

1. Seated Forward Fold (page 130)
2. Seated Twist (page 88)
3. Puppy (page 94)
4. Banana (page 104)
5. Fish (page 108)

## Holding and Repetitions

- Take inhales and exhales that are equal in length. You want to be able to relax into the stretch—but not get so relaxed that you fall back asleep!

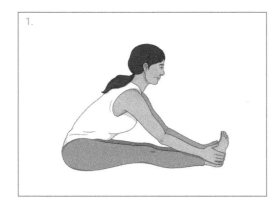

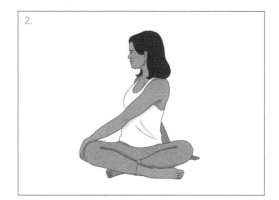

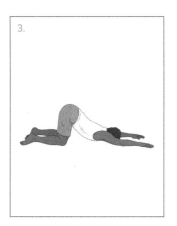

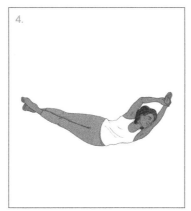

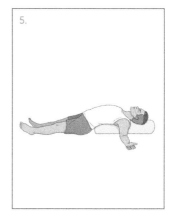

## Remember

- You can do this sequence right in bed each morning to start your day off right. You can use your bed pillows to make each stretch more comfortable.

# EVENING STRETCH

## Good For

- Many people struggle with sleep issues and never think to allow their body to stretch out and physically unwind before bed. This routine will help prepare your body to rest peacefully.

## Routine

1. Child's Pose (page 86)
2. Single Leg Hamstring Stretch (page 142)
3. Single Leg Supine Straddle (page 144)
4. Supine Twist (page 98)
5. Banana (page 104)

## Holding and Repetitions

- Use your breathing to help your mind and body prepare for bed. Inhale for 4 counts, hold for 7 counts, and exhale for 8 counts. Repeat this breathing cycle 3 times during each stretch.

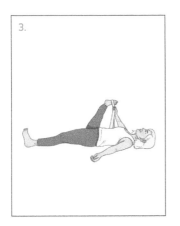

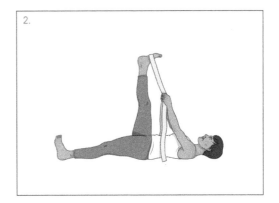

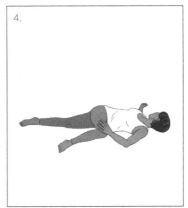

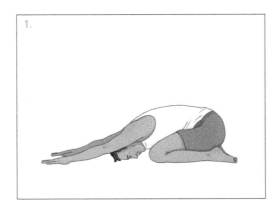

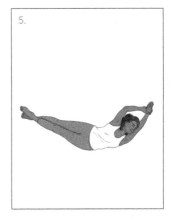

## Remember

- This is another routine that you could do right in bed, so feel free to use pillows to make everything more comfortable.

# MANUAL LABOR

## Good For

- Whether it is moving heavy boxes or doing projects around the house, we really should warm up and prepare the body for activity.

## Routine

1. Arm Swings (page 60)
2. Hip Circles (page 120)
3. Leg Swings (page 152)
4. Standing Side Bend (page 102)
5. Fold with Hands Interlaced (page 56)

## Holding and Repetitions

- Use the dynamic variation for each stretch when possible. Perform for 1 minute in each direction and hold the final stretch for 30 seconds.

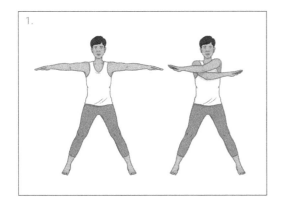

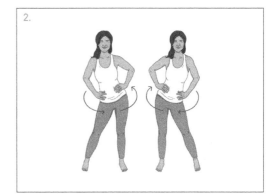

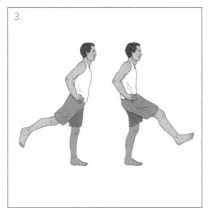

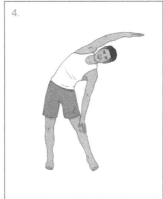

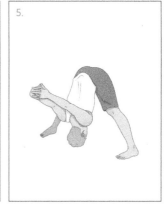

## Remember

- Try to move a little slowly at first to find your full range of motion before you pick up the pace and really get the blood flowing.

# NEW PARENTS

## Good For

- Coming home with a new baby takes a toll on the body in a wide variety of ways, and stretching can really help make a difference.

## Routine

1. Quadruped Cat Cow (page 84) or Seated Cat Cow (page 82)
2. Twisted Twist (page 100)
3. Reclining Pigeon (page 116)
4. Banana (page 104)
5. Child's Pose (page 86)

## Holding and Repetitions

- New parents need a little stress relief and relaxation in as little time as possible! Try using a 4-count inhale and 6-count exhale to help you relax. Repeat this cycle of breathing 6 times during each stretch.

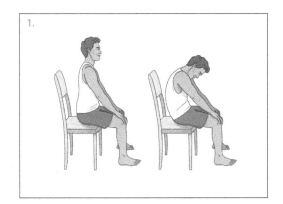

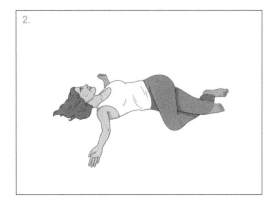

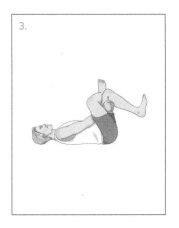

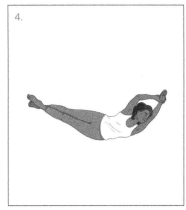

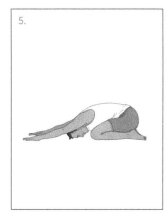

## Remember

- Child's Pose is a restorative posture, so feel free to end here and spend as many minutes in it as you can spare!

# PLAYING WITH KIDS

## Good For

- Playing with kids often happens down on the floor—a place adults don't find very comfortable for sitting or playing. This routine will loosen up the muscles that help you sit down and get up off the floor.

## Routine

1. Butterfly (page 114)
2. Seated Straddle (page 134)
3. Seated Twist (page 88)
4. Reclining Pigeon (page 116)

## Holding and Repetitions

- Hold each stretch for 45 to 60 seconds and repeat the entire routine twice. Use a 4-count inhale and 6-count exhale to help you sink deeper with each exhale.

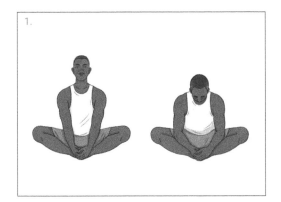

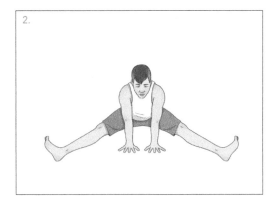

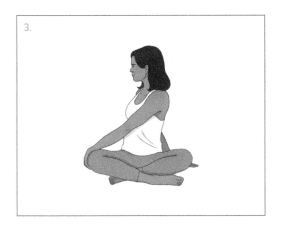

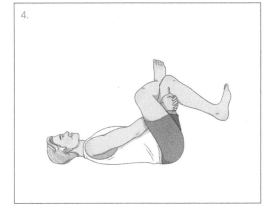

## Remember

- These stretches can be challenging, so be sure to use props to make the stretches more comfortable.

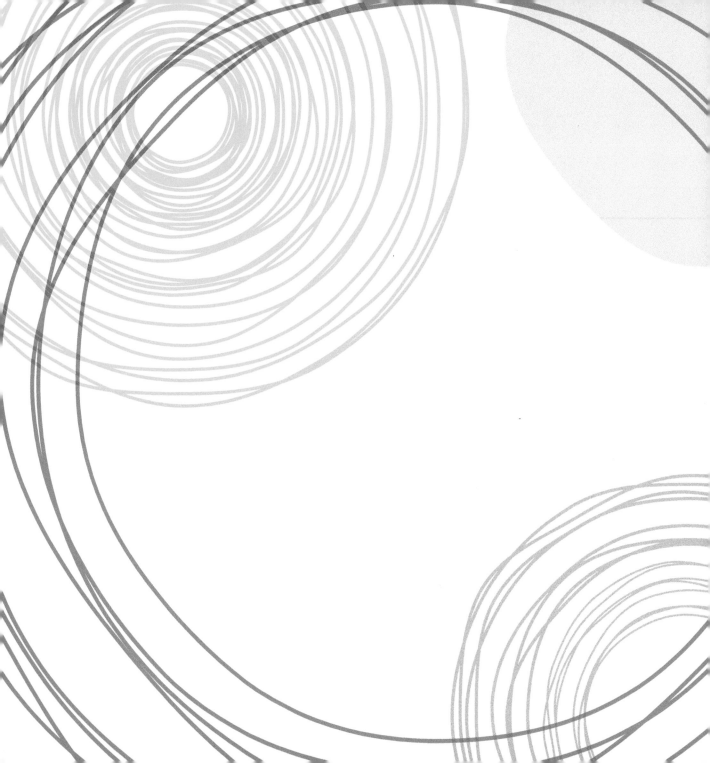

CHAPTER 12

# Active Living

# RUNNING

## Good For

- Running can result in a wide array of minor and major injuries, but this routine will help you recover.

## Routine

1. Standing Quad Stretch (page 126)
2. Runner's Calf Stretch (page 162)
3. IT Band Fold (page 138)
4. Fold with Hands Interlaced (page 56)

## Holding and Repetitions

- You can do all these stretches standing up before you even come inside from your run. Hold each stretch for 1 full minute while slowing your breathing back to normal.

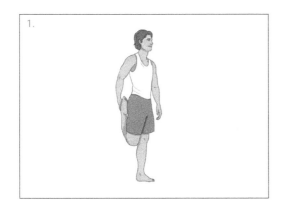

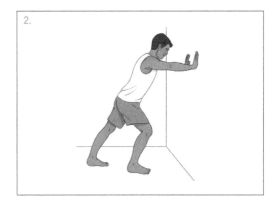

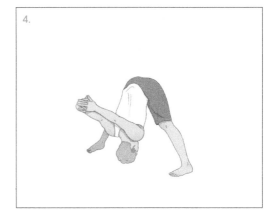

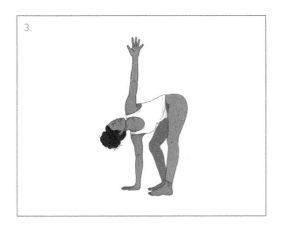

## Remember

- These are all static stretches, so make sure you do this routine after your run and not before. You could do the Walking routine (page 174) instead to prepare for your run.

# CYCLING

## Good For

- This routine can be done before or after you hop on a bike. It will help stretch the quads, hamstrings, hips, shoulders, and chest—an excellent total body stretch!

## Routine

1. Standing Quad Stretch (page 126)
2. Runner's Lunge (page 122)
3. Half Split (page 140)
4. Shoulder Circles (page 50)
5. Back Scratch (page 58)

## Holding and Repetitions

- Hold each stretch for 1 minute on each side using slow, deep breathing.

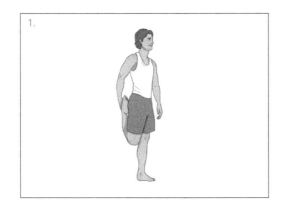

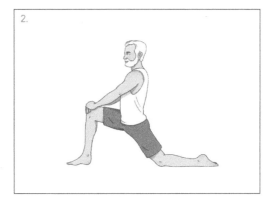

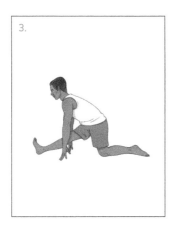

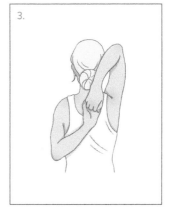

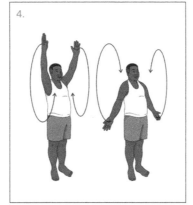

## Remember

- If you are using this routine as a warm-up, continually change sides on the Standing Quad Stretch and then combine the Runner's Lunge and Half Split into a dynamic stretch. moving back and forth from the Runner's Lunge to the Half Split.

# SWIMMING

## Good For

- This is an excellent sequence to prepare the body for any type of swimming. It will help increase the range of motion in your shoulders while also increasing lung capacity.

## Routine

1. Shoulder Circles (page 50)
2. Arm Swings (page 60)
3. Back Scratch (page 58)
4. Fish (page 108)

## Holding and Repetitions

- Do all of the stretches for 1 minute each. Let your breathing naturally sync up to the dynamic movements.

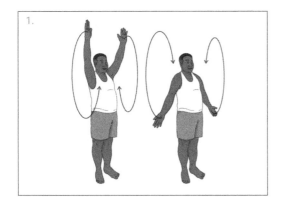

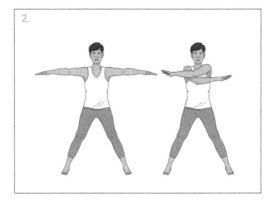

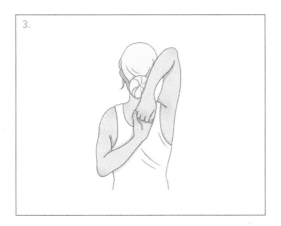

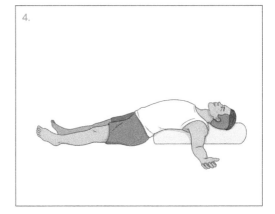

## Remember

- Feel free to hold Fish pose for as long as you can at the end to help improve your lung capacity and reverse rounded shoulders.

# GOLF

## Good For

- This routine will help get your body ready to twist and swing a golf club with mobility and power.

## Routine

1. Shoulder Circles (page 50)
2. Hip Circles (page 120)
3. Cross Body Stretch (page 52)
4. Seated Twist (page 88)

## Holding and Repetitions

- This routine was designed as a warm-up, so you should be continually moving in each dynamic stretch. For the Cross Body Stretch and Seated Twist, continually switch from side to side after a small pause.

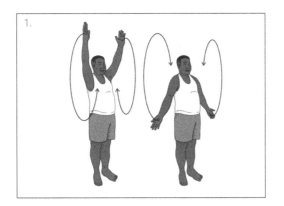

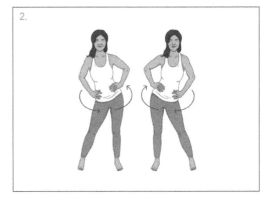

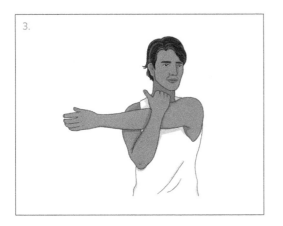

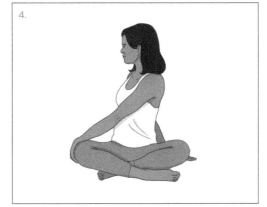

## Remember

- Don't forget to do your Shoulder Circles both forward and backward for 1 minute each. Start with a slow circle to find your full range of motion and then speed up your movement.

# TENNIS/SQUASH

## Good For

- This routine will help prepare the body for any racquet sports like tennis, racquetball, or squash by opening up the shoulder joints and preparing the lower body for quick stops, deep lunges, and pivots.

## Routine

1. Arm Swings (page 60)
2. Cross Body Stretch (page 52)
3. Ankle Circles (page 158)
4. Hip Circles (page 120)
5. Side Lunge (page 132)

## Holding and Repetitions

- Use the dynamic version of each stretch. Perform each stretch for 1 minute and repeat the entire sequence again. Let your breath connect with each movement.

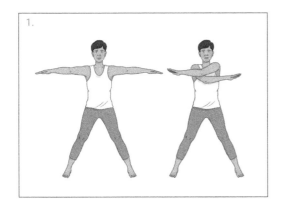

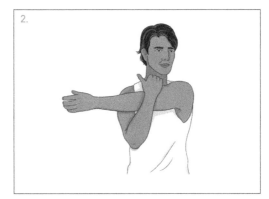

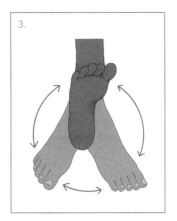

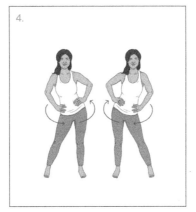

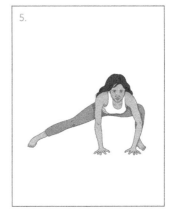

## Remember

- Don't forget to do your circles in clockwise and counterclockwise directions.

# PADDLE SPORTS

## Good For

- This routine will help prepare the upper body and core muscles for paddling activities like kayaking, canoeing, and paddleboarding.

## Routine

1. Arm Swings (page 60)
2. Shoulder Circles (page 50)
3. Hip Circles (page 120)
4. Standing Side Bend (page 102)

## Holding and Repetitions

- Do each exercise for 1 minute and let your breath naturally sync up with the movements. Don't forget to do your circles for 1 minute in each direction. Alternate your dynamic Standing Side Bends from side to side.

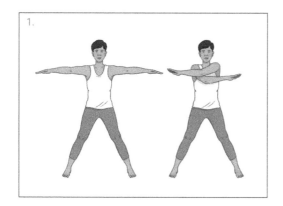

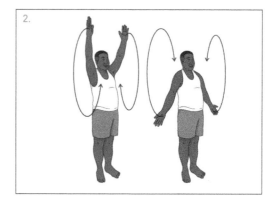

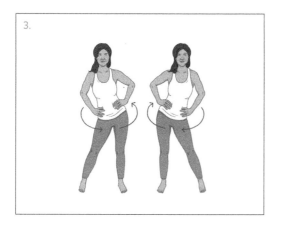

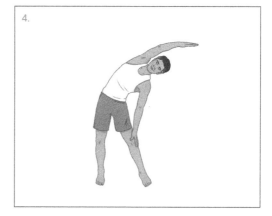

## Remember

- Don't forget to do your circles for 1 minute in each direction. Alternate your dynamic Standing Side Bends from side to side. Do your Arm Swings with the added twisting movement from side to side that is listed in its modifications.

# HIKING

## Good For

- This routine will help prepare the lower body for hiking and walking on hills and rough terrain.

## Routine

1. Ankle Alphabet (page 156)
2. Hip Circles (page 120)
3. Leg Swings (page 152)
4. Standing Quad Stretch (page 126)
5. Runner's Calf Stretch (page 162)

## Holding and Repetitions

- Spend 1 full minute in each stretch while breathing slowly and gently. The Standing Quad Stretch and Runner's Calf Stretch are static stretches, so only hold them for 30 seconds on each side and then repeat one more time.

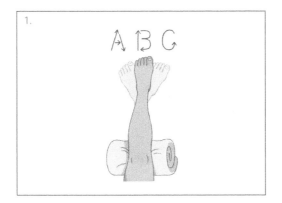

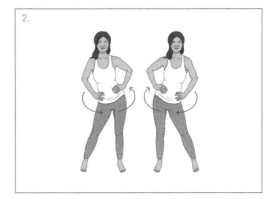

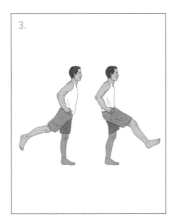

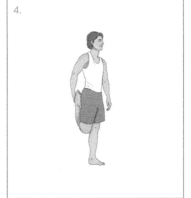

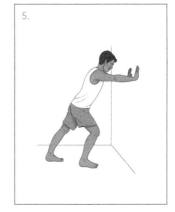

## Remember

- I recommend doing this routine when you get to your hiking destination. You can sit in your car to do the Ankle Alphabet and do the rest of the stretches standing outside.

# WEIGHT LIFTING

## Good For

- It is important to prepare the body to lift weights. This routine is a total body warm-up that will help you get the blood flowing to all the major muscles.

## Routine

1. Shoulder Circles (page 50)
2. Leg Swings (page 152)
3. Standing Side Bend (page 102)
4. Torso Extension with Countertop (page 110)

## Holding and Repetitions

- Perform each stretch for 1 minute on each side while allowing your breath to connect with the movement. The last stretch is not dynamic, so hold it for about 30 seconds and release.

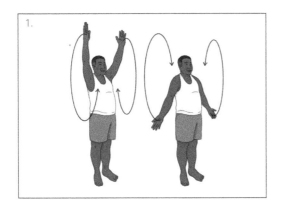

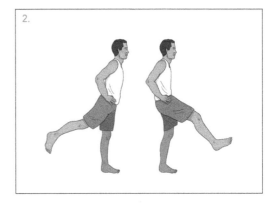

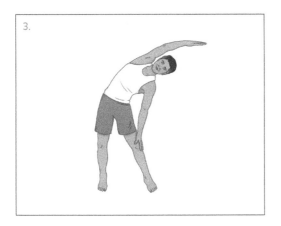

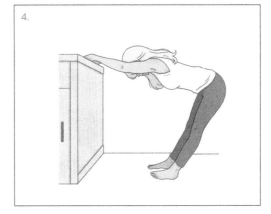

## Remember

- You may not be able to find a countertop at the gym, but there are many different pieces of equipment you can use to hold on to instead. Just make sure that whatever you're holding on to is very sturdy.

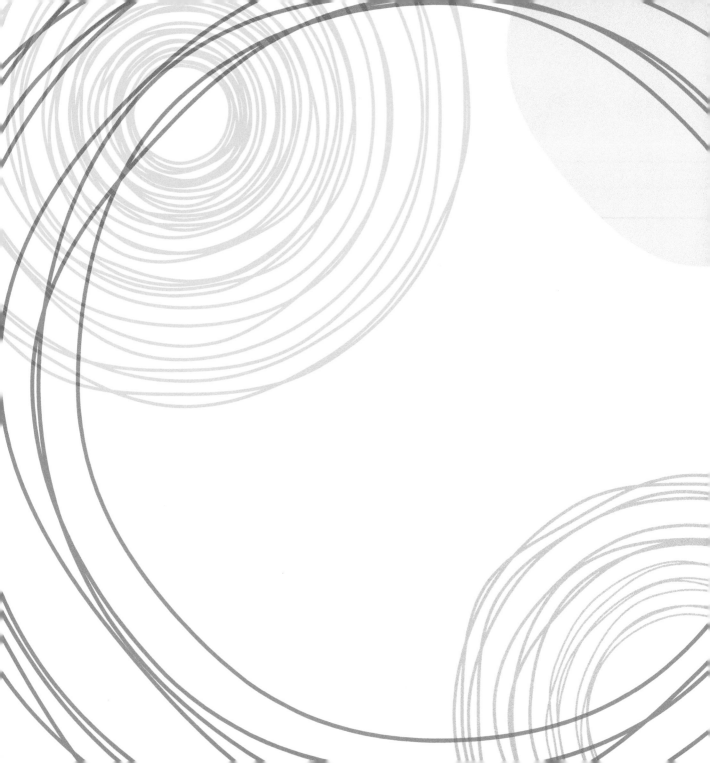

CHAPTER 13

# Injury Recovery

# SPRAINED ANKLE

## Good For

- All ankle injuries could benefit from these stretches. The Ankle Alphabet also helps stretch and strengthen the ankle joint.

## Routine

1. Point and Flex (page 148)
2. Ankle Circles (page 158)
3. Ankle Alphabet (page 156)
4. Towel Pulls (page 150)

## Holding and Repetitions

- Take your time and move very slowly in each movement for 1 minute. Let your breath connect with the movement or try a 4-count inhale and 6-count exhale to help with pain.

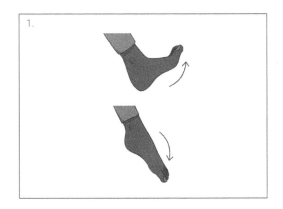

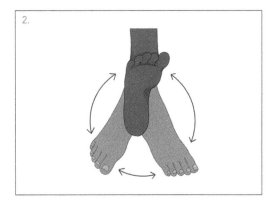

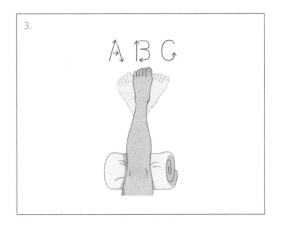

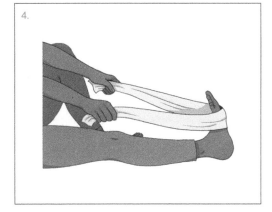

## Remember

- I always recommend that my clients do both ankles and not just the injured side. It is important to take care of both ankles because your healthy ankle compensates for the injured side.

# SHOULDER PAIN

## Good For

- This sequence can address a wide array of shoulder issues by helping to gently stretch the surrounding muscles.

## Routine

1. Stir the Pot (page 66)
2. Cross Body Stretch (page 52)
3. Doorway Pec Stretch (page 106)
4. Back Scratch (page 58)

## Holding and Repetitions

- Let your pain guide how long you hold the stretches. Try to get to 1 full minute, even if that means repeating the stretch 3 times for 20 seconds.

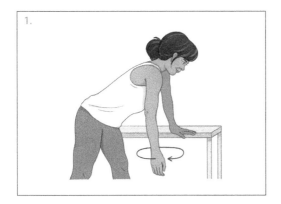

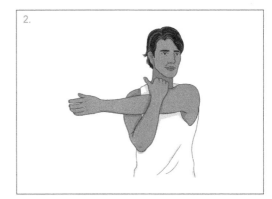

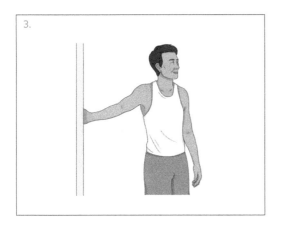

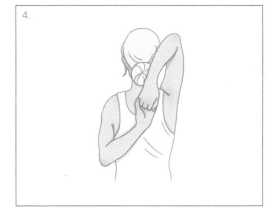

## Remember

- Don't forget to Stir the Pot in both directions. You can also hold the Doorway Pec Stretch at a variety of different heights to hit the exact spot you need.

# HIP REPLACEMENT

## Good For

- This routine could be helpful for hip pain, bursitis, arthritis, or before or after a hip replacement.

## Routine

1. Standing Straddle (page 136)

2. Hip Circles (page 120)

3. Twisted Twist (page 100)

4. Reclining Pigeon (page 116)

5. Supine Twist (page 98)

## Holding and Repetitions

- Hold each stretch for 1 full minute while using a 4-count inhale and 6-count exhale.

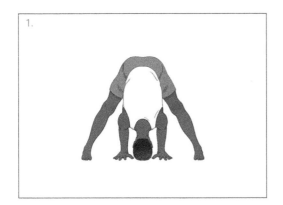

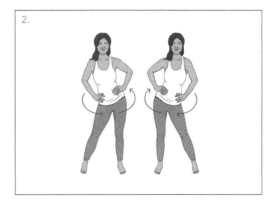

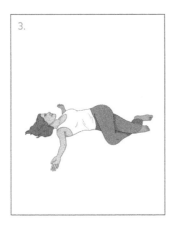

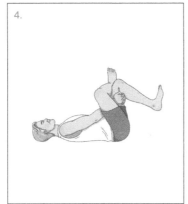

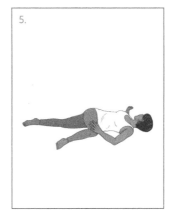

## Remember

- Use pillows under your knees to help keep your body as supported as possible in each stretch. Remember, the pillows are not cheating; rather, they are a way to help your body get more out of the stretch.

# HAMSTRING STRAIN

## Good For

- You have to be gentle when stretching a hamstring strain, as it has already stretched too much. These stretches will help the surrounding muscles in addition to engaging and stretching the hamstring itself.

## Routine

1. Runner's Calf Stretch (page 162)
2. Runner's Lunge (page 122)
3. Hurdler's Stretch (page 118)
4. Single Leg Hamstring Stretch (page 142)

## Holding and Repetitions

- Hold each stretch for 1 full minute while using a 4-count inhale and 6-count exhale.

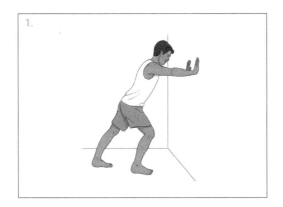

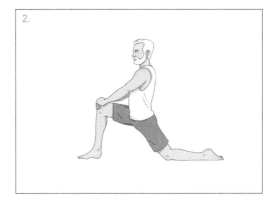

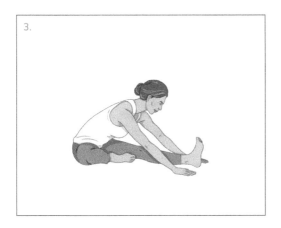

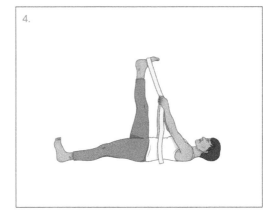

## Remember

- Use the active version of the Runner's Lunge by lifting your back knee off the floor so the hamstring muscle can fully engage.

# KNEE REHAB

## Good For

- Whether you have IT band, ACL, or MCL issues, or have had knee reconstruction or a knee replacement, these stretches will help reduce tension in the surrounding muscles.

## Routine

1. Standing Quad Stretch (page 126)
2. IT Band Fold (page 138)
3. Hurdler's Stretch (page 118)
4. Supine Twist (page 98)

## Holding and Repetitions

- Hold each stretch for 1 minute on each side while using a 4-count inhale and 6-count exhale.

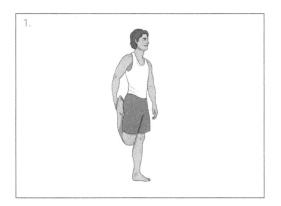

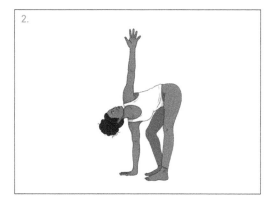

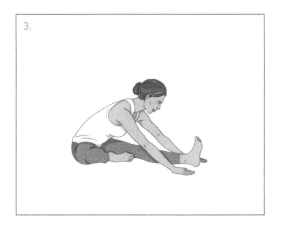

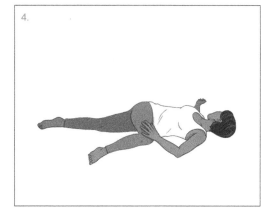

## Remember

- You can place a pillow under your knee to make each stretch more comfortable. For the Standing Quad Stretch, you can place a pillow on a chair and rest your knee there while you use a towel to help pull your foot into the stretch.

# PLANTAR FASCIITIS

## Good For

- Heel pain and plantar fasciitis are often caused by tightness and restrictions in the calf muscle, which makes stretching an effective treatment modality in many cases.

## Routine

1. Runner's Calf Stretch (page 162)
2. Wall Calf Stretch (page 160)
3. Towel Pulls (page 150)
4. Ankle Circles (page 158)

## Holding and Repetitions

- Perform each stretch for 1 minute on each side and make sure you do the Ankle Circles for 1 minute in each direction. Breathe slowly and gently throughout each stretch.

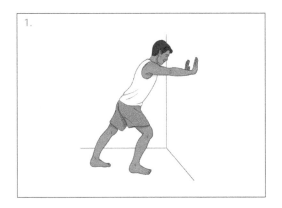

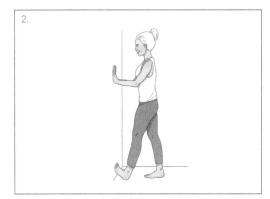

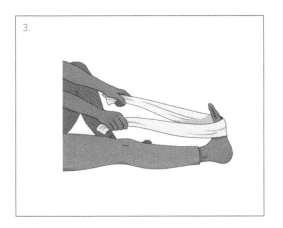

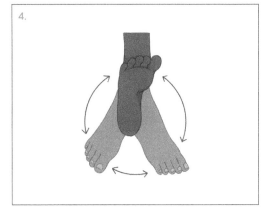

## Remember

- Although this pain usually affects just one side, make sure you do the stretches on both sides. This will allow your body to come into better balance with every step you take after your stretch session.

# SHIN SPLINTS

## Good For

- Shin splints are an unnecessary but common source of pain for many runners and athletes. This routine will help prevent them and treat them.

## Routine

1. Ankle Alphabet (page 156)
2. Towel Pulls (page 150)
3. Standing Quad Stretch (page 126)
4. Runner's Calf Stretch (page 162)

## Holding and Repetitions

- Spend 1 minute on each stretch. Use a slow, gentle breath while doing the Ankle Alphabet, and switch over to a 4-count inhale and 6-count exhale as you do the other stretches.

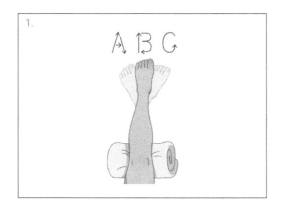

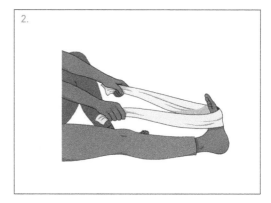

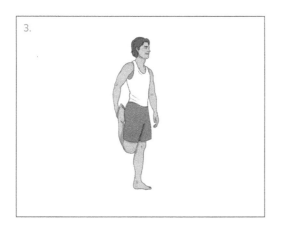

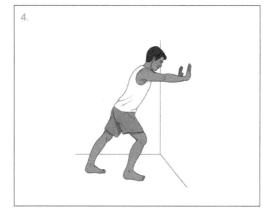

## Remember

- If you are using this routine as a warm-up before you run, hold the standing stretches for 30 seconds on each side and then repeat on each side.

# GROIN PULL

## Good For

- Groin pain can stem from tight, weak, pulled, or strained muscles but can be resolved by gently stretching the surrounding muscles.

## Routine

1. Hip Circles (page 120)
2. Runner's Lunge (page 122)
3. Butterfly (page 114)
4. Seated Straddle (page 134)

## Holding and Repetitions

- Spend 1 minute in each stretch while using a 4-count inhale and 6-count exhale. In the Seated Straddle, spend 1 minute reaching toward each leg and reaching to the middle.

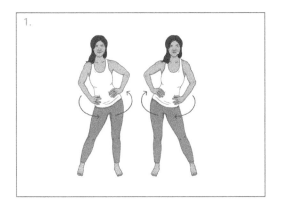

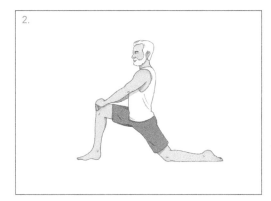

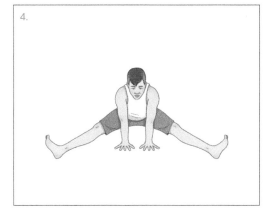

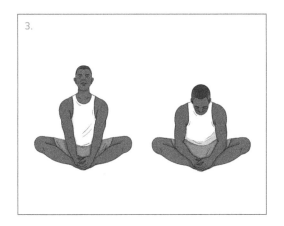

## Remember

- You don't have to go into your deepest stretch to get the benefits. If you are experiencing any pain, back out of the stretch a little bit and hold it there instead.

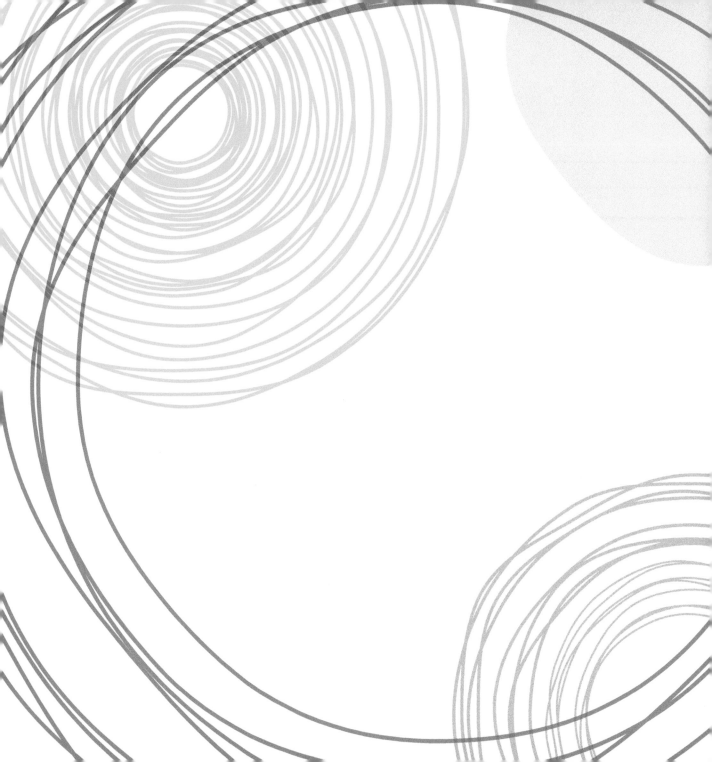

# Aches and Pains

# SCIATICA PAIN

## Good For

- Sciatica pain is often caused by an accumulation of tension within the gluteus muscles, lower back, and hips, so this stretching routine can provide a great deal of relief.

## Routine

1. Hip Circles (page 120)
2. Single Leg Hamstring Stretch (page 142)
3. Supine Twist (page 98)
4. Banana (page 104)
5. Reclining Pigeon (page 116)

## Holding and Repetitions

- Spend 1 minute in each stretch using the 5-count box breathing technique (page x) or a 4-count inhale and 6-count exhale.

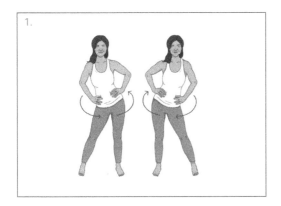

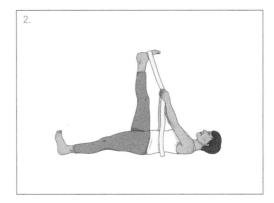

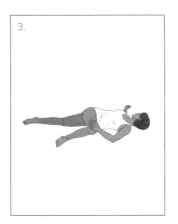

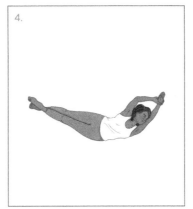

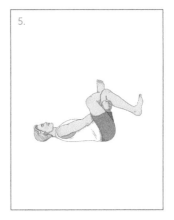

## Remember

- Pause after each stretch and let your body return to a resting position. Notice which stretch provides the greatest pain relief so you will remember to use it in times of need.

# STIFF NECK

## Good For

- Waking up with a stiff neck is never a pleasant surprise. Use these stretches to help get your neck moving normally again.

## Routine

1. Head Nods (page 38)
2. Head Turns (page 36)
3. Half Circles (page 42)
4. Ear to Shoulder (page 40)

## Holding and Repetitions

- Do each stretch for 1 full minute and repeat the entire sequence again. If your neck is too tender to hold for a minute, try holding for 30 seconds and repeating the sequence 4 times.

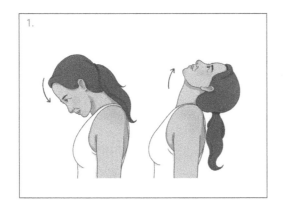

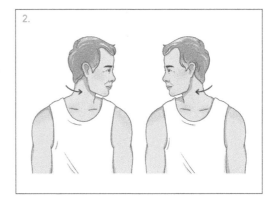

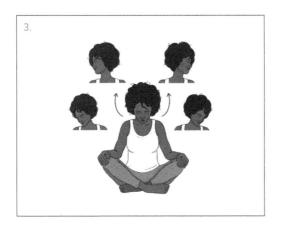

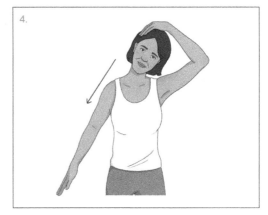

## Remember

- Your neck muscles can be very tender, so be sure to move very slowly. You can actually pretend you have to move as slowly as humanly possible, and you may get even more out of the stretch!

# LOWER BACK PAIN

## Good For

- Lower back pain isn't always caused by the lower back itself. This routine will help stretch all the muscles that can contribute to lower back pain.

## Routine

1. Quadruped Cat Cow (page 84) or Seated Cat Cow (page 82)
2. Runner's Lunge (page 122)
3. Twisted Twist (page 100)
4. Reclining Pigeon (page 116)

## Holding and Repetitions

- Spend 1 minute in each stretch, on each side. Use a 4-count inhale and 6-count exhale to help decrease your pain levels as you relax deeper into each stretch.

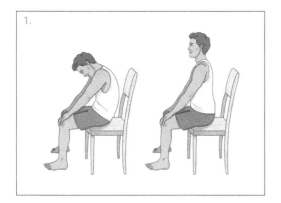

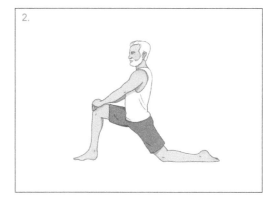

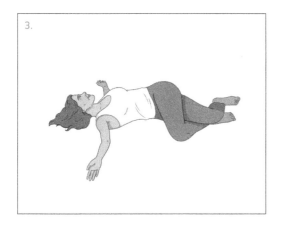

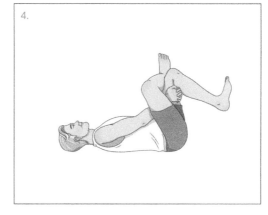

## Remember

- Don't forget to do the Twisted Twist for 1 minute to the left and to the right before you cross your legs the opposite way.

# HAND AND WRIST ISSUES

## Good For

- Pain can arise in the fingers, hands, and wrists due to carpal tunnel syndrome or arthritis, but these exercises will help create more synovial fluid in the joints while stretching the surrounding muscles.

## Routine

1. Finger Spread (page 78)
2. Wrist Extension (page 74)
3. Wrist Flexion (page 72)
4. Hand and Knees Wrist Circles (page 76)
5. Wrist Roll Out (page 70)

## Holding and Repetitions

- Spend 1 minute in each stretch using slow and gentle breathing. Take your time and move slowly while keeping the rest of your body as relaxed as possible.

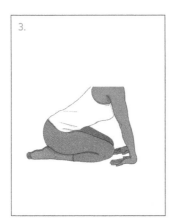

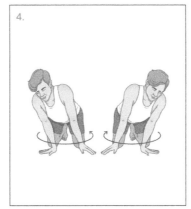

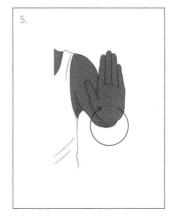

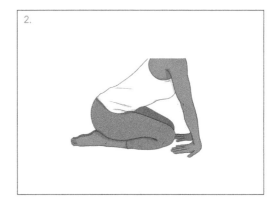

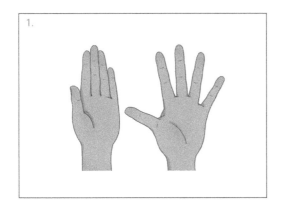

## Remember

- You can place your hands on a table instead of getting down on the floor, which can help you take more weight and pressure off the wrists if necessary.

# HEADACHE

## Good For

- Many times headaches are caused by an accumulation of stress and tension. The natural remedy is to drink a glass of water, take some deep breaths, and do the following routine!

## Routine

1. Head Turns (page 36)
2. Ear to Shoulder (page 40)
3. Half Circles (page 42)
4. Shoulder Shrug and Release (page 48)

## Holding and Repetitions

- Allow your head to move slowly in each stretch for 1 minute each while using a 4-count inhale and 6-count exhale. If you want, repeat the routine for a second time for a total of 10 minutes.

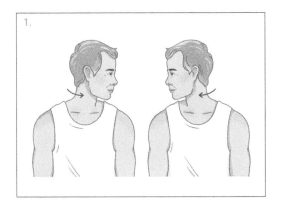

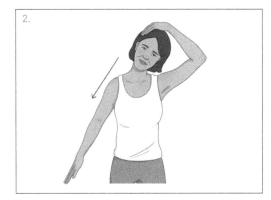

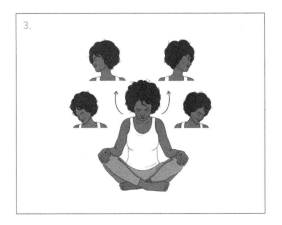

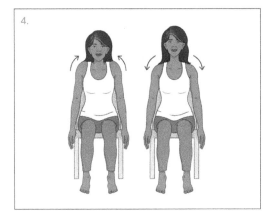

## Remember

- You can do all of these stretches while relaxing on the couch. Make this routine as comfortable as possible to help eliminate your headache.

# KNEE PAIN

## Good For

- Knee pain is often caused by tight IT bands or quadricep muscles. This routine will help you identify what muscles may be contributing to your knee pain while stretching all the surrounding muscles.

## Routine

1. Standing Quad Stretch (page 126)
2. IT Band Fold (page 138)
3. Runner's Lunge (page 122)
4. Half Split (page 140)

## Holding and Repetitions

- Hold each stretch for 1 minute on each side while using a 4-count inhale and 6-count exhale.

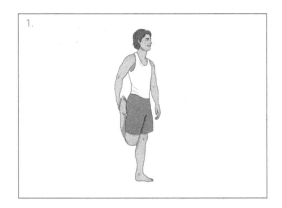

1.

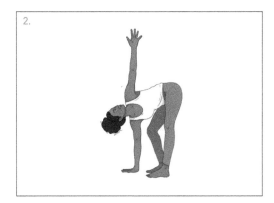

2.

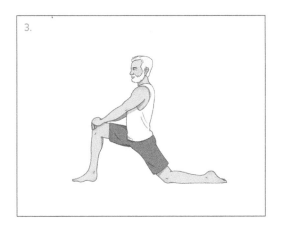

3.

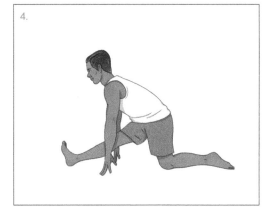

4.

## Remember

- Make sure you use props to make this routine more comfortable. I highly recommend using a chair on each side of you to help you balance and placing a pillow under your knee for the Runner's Lunge and Half Split.

# ELBOW PAIN

## Good For

- Repetitive use of the elbow can lead to strain, often referred to as tennis elbow or golfer's elbow depending on which side the pain is located. Stretching and ice is generally the best method of healing.

## Routine

1. Ear to Shoulder (page 40)
2. Cross Body Stretch (page 52)
3. Back Scratch (page 58)
4. Wrist Flexion (page 72)
5. Wrist Extension (page 74)
6. Hand and Knees Wrist Circles (page 76)

## Holding and Repetitions

- Hold each stretch for 1 minute on each side or moving in each direction while using a 4-count inhale and 6-count exhale.

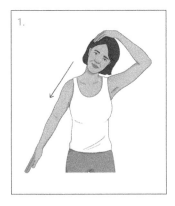

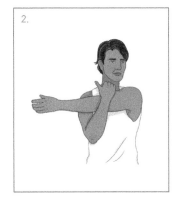

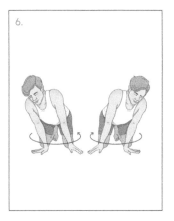

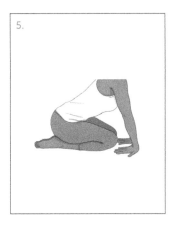

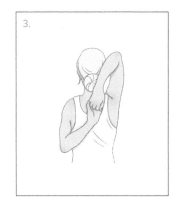

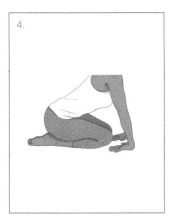

## Remember

- Move slowly and if anything causes pain, stop completely or try a much smaller movement.

# HIP PAIN

## Good For

- This routine should open up your hips at every single angle to help diminish pain in the hips and glutes.

## Routine

1. Hip Circles (page 120)
2. Runner's Lunge (page 122)
3. Butterfly (page 114)
4. Reclining Pigeon (page 116)

## Holding and Repetitions

- Hold each stretch for 1 minute using a 4-count inhale and 6-count exhale. Use two different leg variations in Butterfly pose for 1 minute each.

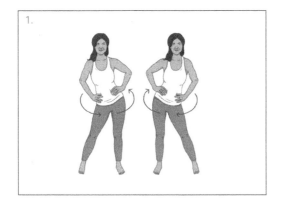

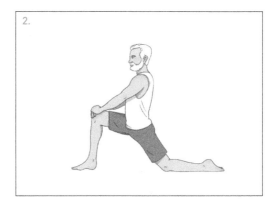

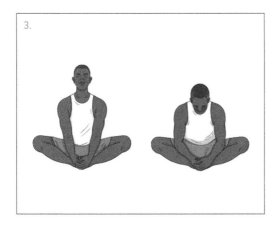

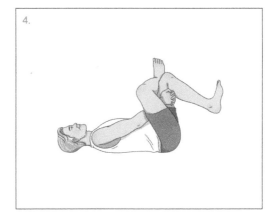

## Remember

- Create a stronger mind and body connection by taking the time to connect with your hip pain in each stretch. Imagine sending your inhales into the pain and, as you exhale, the pain leaving the body with your breath.

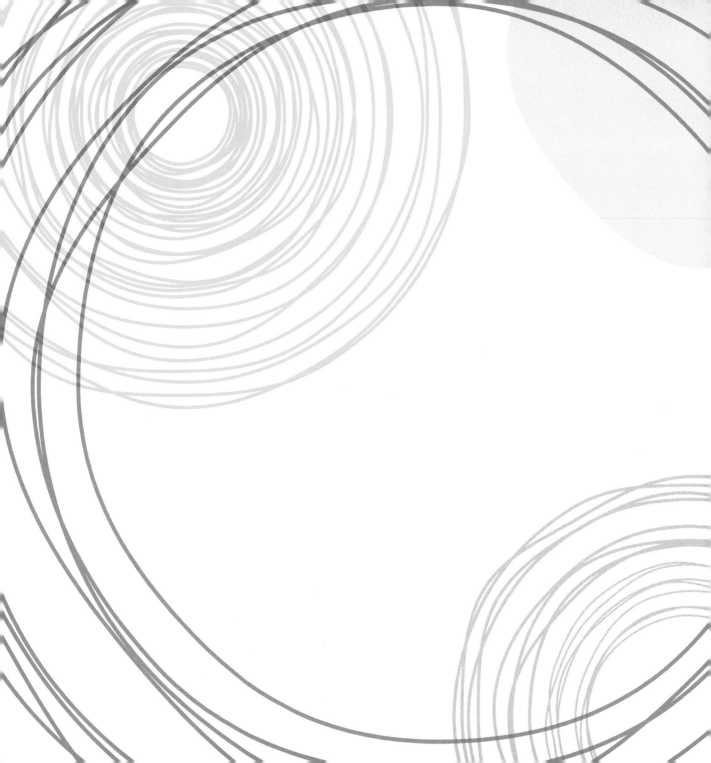

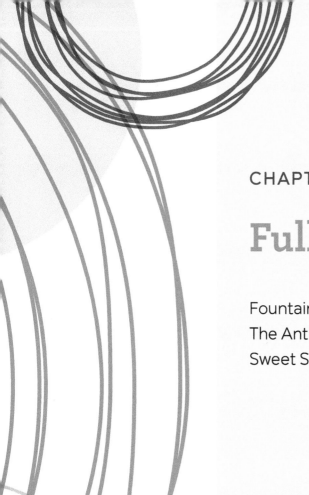

CHAPTER 15

# Full Body Release

# FOUNTAIN OF YOUTH

## Good For

- Our spine can move and bend in six different directions, and they say the healthier our spine is, the younger we feel! This sequence will help improve your spinal health and overall mobility.

## Routine

1. Seated Forward Fold (page 130)
2. Fish (page 108)
3. Supine Twist (page 98)
4. Banana (page 104)

## Holding and Repetitions

- Hold each stretch for 90 seconds while using the 5-count box breathing technique (page x).

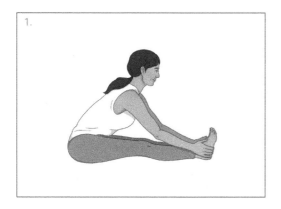

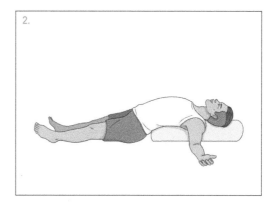

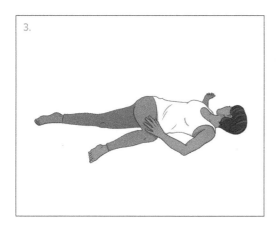

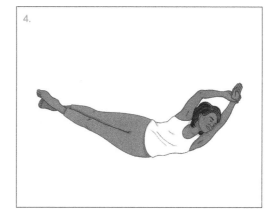

## Remember

- Think about your spine in each stretch by bringing your awareness to the base of your spine and trying to create more length from the tailbone to the crown of your head.

# THE ANTI-DEPRESSANT

## Good For

- Stretching exercises that increase the blood flow to the brain are known for their ability to relieve stress and boost your mood.

## Routine

1. Standing Forward Fold (page 128)
2. Quadruped Cat Cow (page 84) or Seated Cat Cow (page 82)
3. Puppy (page 94)
4. Inverted V (page 166)

## Holding and Repetitions

- This is a slower practice with a 2-minute hold for each stretch. The Cat Cow is a dynamic stretch, but feel free to hold in each phase for any length that feels right.

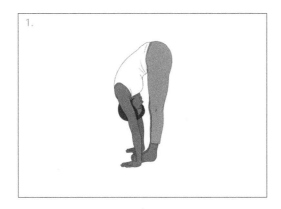

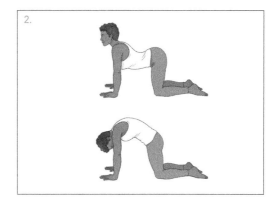

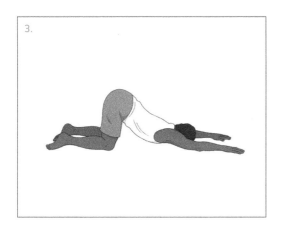

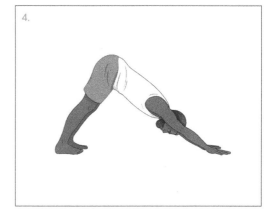

## Remember

- The blood does rush to your head in some of these positions more than others. Take your time as you are transitioning out of each stretch so the change in blood pressure doesn't make you lightheaded.

# SWEET SURRENDER

## Good For

- This sequence helps the spine relax by bending and twisting it in different directions. Once the muscles of the spine relax, your entire body will soften and surrender.

## Routine

1. Child's Pose (page 86)
2. Reclining Pigeon (page 116)
3. Supine Twist (page 98)
4. Banana (page 104)

## Holding and Repetitions

- Use a 4-count inhale and 6-count exhale during each stretch. Take 9 of these breaths in each position.

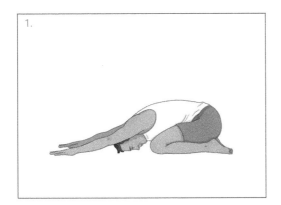

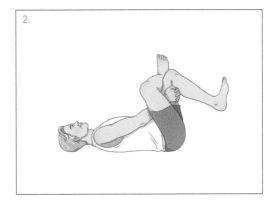

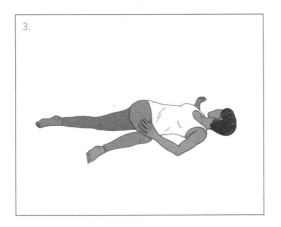

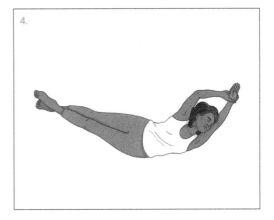

## Remember

- Remain focused on your breathing to help your mind relax. This is the perfect routine to do right in bed at night.

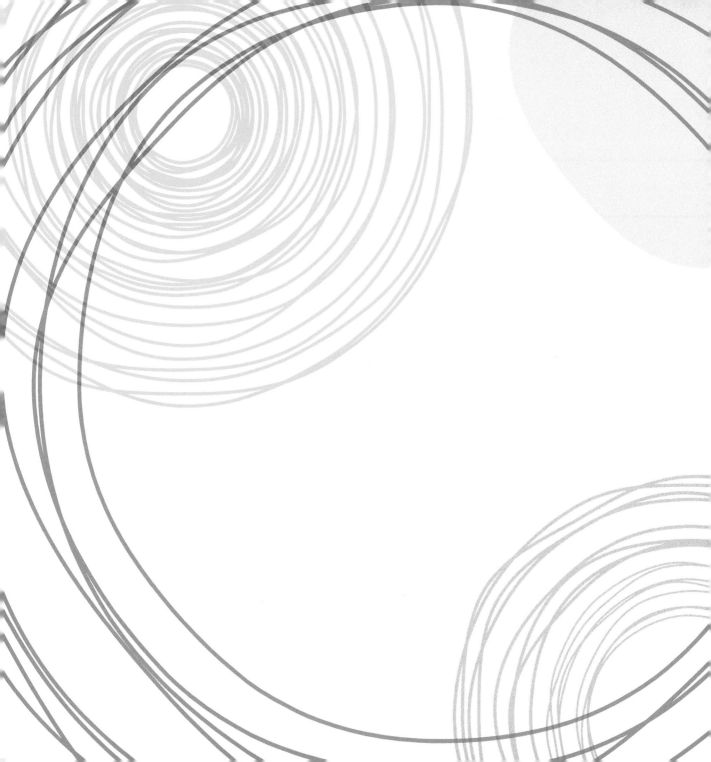

CHAPTER 16

# Customize Your Stretching Practice

Once you have tried out all of the sequences in this book, it's time to start creating your own routines! I recommend getting very familiar with all the stretches and routines in the book so you have firsthand knowledge of how the stretches feel in your body and which ones you need the most. This will help you create a customized routine for yourself.

# What Makes a Good—and Safe—Stretching Routine?

Everything I have taught you about stretching should ensure that you are able to create a safe and effective stretching routine, but these are the five most important things to keep in mind:

1. Start with dynamic stretches to get the body warmed up. If you are doing a stretch routine after other activities, then this isn't a concern and isn't mandatory.

2. Choose stretches that feel good in your body. Don't just pick out your least favorite stretches and make a routine with them! Make sure you have a balance of stretches that are challenging and enjoyable. Keep your personal limitations in mind, and don't use any stretches that cause pain.

3. Experiment with different variations of each stretch. Try making it an active, dynamic, static, or PNF stretch to find which approach provides the best results in your body. Everyone is unique!

4. Play with the order of the stretches. I know how to create the perfect order of stretches to achieve different benefits, but you may not have that expertise. Once you select the stretches you want in your routine, try doing them in a different order each time until you find the best combination.

5. Don't forget to connect with your breath. Try different breathing techniques to see what works best in the sequence you have created. It may be mindful breathing, box breathing (page x), a 4-count inhale and 6-count exhale, or just focusing on a slow exhale.

# Try This

When you are creating a new routine, there are a couple of different methods I recommend for keeping track of them. If you are a pen and paper person, start a little stretching journal to keep track of your sessions. When creating a new routine, give it a name and write down the names of the stretches it includes, as well as the corresponding page numbers in this book, for reference. If you tend to use technology more than pen and paper, you can do this on your phone. A handy way to do this with your phone is to take photos of the illustrations for each stretch and make a photo album of your stretch routine.

Here are three ideas to help you start thinking about how to create a sequence:

- Idea 1: Choose two dynamic stretches and two static stretches.

- Idea 2: Choose one upper body, one torso, and one lower body stretch.

- Idea 3: Put all the standing stretches together.

Get the idea? Think about the sequences you did in the book and which ones felt best in your body. This is why it can be helpful to keep a stretching journal. Stretching also has psychological, emotional, and spiritual benefits, so keeping a journal may help you connect with insights you have while stretching or recognize emotional shifts that occur. Keeping notes about your favorite sessions can inspire you to create new routines by combining some of your favorites in different ways. No matter what sequences you invent, make sure to move slowly and listen to your body. Take your time and don't forget to connect with your breathing.

# Resources

If you would like to continue your education further, these are go-to resources for information on safe stretching and how to better care for your body.

## Websites and Apps

The Flexibility Guru: My own website includes a full video library of individual stretches, stretch routines, and workouts at TheFlexibilityGuru.com.

Gold Medal Bodies: This site offers online training programs with gymnastics-based mobility workouts at GMB.io.

StretchIt App: Available on the App Store and Google Play or on the web, this app offers video stretching classes right on your device. Look them up at StretchItApp.com.

## Books

*Resistance Flexibility 1.0: Becoming Flexible in All Ways* by Bob Cooley

*The Roll Model: A Step-by-Step Guide to Erase Pain, Improve Mobility, and Live Better in Your Body* by Jill Miller

*1,500 Stretches: The Complete Guide to Flexibility and Movement* by Hollis Liebman

*Becoming a Supple Leopard* by Kelly Starrett with Glen Cardoza

*Tight Hip, Twisted Core: The Key to Unresolved Pain* by Christine Koth

*The Vital Psoas Muscle: Connecting Physical, Emotional, and Spiritual Well-Being* by Jo Ann Staugaard-Jones

*The Complete Illustrated Book of Yoga* by Swami Vishnudevananda

*Yoga Toolbox for Teachers and Students* by Joseph and Lillian Le Page

# References

Cooley, Bob. *Resistance Flexibility 1.0: Becoming Flexible in All Ways*. Dublin, OH: Telemachus Press, LLC, 2016.

Fried, Linda P., Nemat O. Borhani, et al. "The Cardiovascular Health Study: Design And Rationale". *Annals Of Epidemiology*, 1, no. 3 (1991): 263-276 . doi:10.1016/1047-2797 (91)90005-w.

Gergley, Jeffery C. "Acute Effect of Passive Static Stretching on Lower-Body Strength in Moderately Trained Men." *The Journal of Strength and Conditioning Research* 27, no. 4. (April 2013): 973–977. DOI:10.1519/JSC.0b013e318260b7ce.

Horovitz, Bruce. "Decade by Decade, Aging Presents Common Challenges." *MedicalXpress*. April 12, 2018. MedicalXpress.com/news/2018-04-decade-aging-common.html.

Nierenberg, Cari. "Is 90 the New 80? Most 90-Somethings Feel Healthy." *LiveScience*. March 20, 2017. LiveScience.com/58333-90-somethings-feel-healthy.html.

Nojiri, Shusuke, Masahide Yagi, Yu Mizukami, and Noriyaki Ichihashi. "Static Stretching Time Required to Reduce Iliacus Muscle Stiffness." *Sports Biomechanics* (June 2019): 1–10. DOI:10.1080/14763141.2019.1620321.

Thomas, Ewan; Antonino Bianco; Antonio Paoli; and Antonio Palma. "The Relation Between Stretching Typology and Stretching Duration: The Effects on Range of Motion." *International Journal of Sports Medicine* 39, no. 4 (April 2018): 243–254. DOI:10.1055/s-0044-101146.

"Your Health Through The Decades," Harvard Health, September 2018. https://www.health .harvard.edu/staying-healthy/your-health-through-the-decades.

# Index

# Acknowledgments

I am extremely grateful for the many people in my life who have made this book possible. I instantly think of my mentor Kam Thye Chow, and although I miss him dearly, I hope his knowledge continues on through me and we continue helping people feel their best. I also want to thank the amazing clients I have had throughout the years. I have learned so much from you that helped me write this book.

Thank you to my loving partner, Roberto Parada. You were supportive from the start and never complained, regardless of how much time I was glued to my laptop working on this book!

I'm immensely grateful for everyone in my life who holds me up with their support and love, including Nancy and Jerry Hammond, Marcus DeFlorimonte, Veronica Gorlovsky, and Clancy Heicher.

Thank you to my amazing wellness practitioners, Emily Greenstein and Eric Dermond. Your constant support and guidance on my journey through illness is more meaningful than you may ever know.

I owe an enormous debt of gratitude to the entire Callisto publishing team. This book has been an absolute pleasure to write, and I have had an amazing experience, from my first meeting with Joe Cho to working with my editors Andrea Leptinsky, Lorraine Coffey, and Mo Mozuch.

Last but certainly not least, I can't leave out my dog Bodhi. You were by my side throughout this book with your little soothing snores. Thank you for being my loyal sidekick!

# About the Author

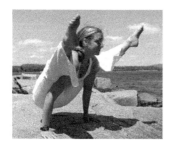 **Hilery Hutchinson** is a wellness expert with over 50 certifications who has spent the past 18 years dedicated to helping people feel their best. She has traveled around the world teaching classes, certifications, and workshops but has finally planted roots in Boston, Massachusetts, while seeing clients worldwide through virtual platforms. She has created several online courses and an on-demand video library that covers many different aspects of fitness and wellness. Hilery loves to go through a thorough assessment process to deeply listen and connect with her clients before she combines all of her knowledge to create a truly customized plan. She wants to improve her clients' quality of life. Her own personal journey through illness has helped her dive even deeper into wellness, self-care, and healing, which has allowed her to help her clients on a deeper level too. To learn more, please visit TheFlexibilityGuru.com.

OCT 2 8 2021

CPSIA information can be obtained
at www.ICGtesting.com
Printed in the USA
JSHW050514260321
12914JS00004B/9